Computer and Template Assisted Orthopedic Surgery

Rolf Haaker
Werner Konerman (Eds.)

Computer and Template Assisted Orthopedic Surgery

With 210 images

Springer

Editors
Haaker, Rolf, Prof. Dr. med.
St. Vincent Hospital
Danziger Str. 17
33034 Brakel

Konermann, Werner, Prof. Dr. med.
Kassel Red Cross Hospital
Hansteinstr. 29
34121 Kassel

ISBN 978-3-642-29727-4 ISBN 978-3-642-29728-1 (eBook)
DOI 10.1007/978-3-642-29728-1

Springer Medizin

Library of Congress Control Number: 2013933370

Editor: Diana Kraplow, Heidelberg
Project Management: Dr. Astrid Horlacher, Heidelberg
Copyediting: Isabella Athanassiou, Bonn
Cover Illustration: © Prof. Dr. Haaker, privat
Cover Design: deblik Berlin
Typesetting and reproduction of the figures: Fotosatz-Service Köhler GmbH – Reinhold Schöberl, Würzburg

Printed on acid-free paper

Springer Medizin is brand of Springer
Springer is part of Springer Science+Business Media (www.springer.com)

Preface

The continued and growing interest in computer-assisted orthopedic surgery (CAOS) prompted us to add a new edition to the two previous volumes on this subject last edited in 2007 by J.B. Stiehl, A.M. DiGioia, and us both.

Moreover, additional developments in the field of CAOS have closed the circle from the methods presented in our first edition in 2001 to the presently available techniques of leg axis restoration and implant positioning by individual cutting devices, as described initially by Portheine and coworkers in the first edition, giving us another reason to do so.

This volume is a combination of the two previous editions. On the one hand, it describes the techniques and initial results of the new methods, which are based on CT or MRI scans of knee joints to prepare patient-individual cutting blocs in external laboratories using the rapid recovery protocol as well as individual implants. On the other hand, this edition illustrates the advances in navigation systems as they »come of age« and become more precise and easier to use.

Last but not least, we give an overview of the use of three-dimensional fluoroscopic devices in the operating theater for the treatment of trauma cases – individually as well as in combination. One chapter in the volume deals with the opportunities of modern robotics in orthopedic surgery.

The last four chapters in particular demonstrate the evolution of computer applications, which will revolutionize the way we perform our surgeries for the next few decades. All the strategies demonstrated here have the same goal: to improve implant positioning along with preservation of soft tissues so as to get better clinical results and increased implant longevity. We hope you enjoy reading about the bases of these techniques and their current applications.

The Editors
Prof. Dr. Rolf G. Haaker
Prof. Dr. Werner Konermann
April 2013

Contents

List of Contributors

Ahmed, Gaffar, MD
Department of Orthopedic Surgery
University Clinic of Giessen and Marburg
Klinikstr. 33
35392 Gießen

Anderl, Werner, Dr.
Barmherzige Schwestern Hospital
Stumpergasse 13
1060 Vienna

Bäthis, Holger, PD Dr.
Department of Orthopedics, Trauma Surgery, and Sports Medicine
Cologne-Merheim Clinic
Ostmerheimer Str. 200
51109 Cologne

Blessing, Recha
University Medical Center
Johannes Gutenberg University of Mainz
II Medical Clinic
Langenbeckstr. 1
55131 Mainz

Botimer, Gary D., MD
Loma Linda University Medical Center
11370 Anderson Street, Suite 1500
Loma Linda 92354, CA, USA

Calliess, Tilman, Dr.
Department of Orthopedic Surgery, Annastift Hospital
Hannover Medical School
Anna-von-Borries-Str. 1–7
30625 Hannover

Citak, Musa, PD Dr.
Department of Trauma Surgery
Hannover Medical School
Carl-Neuberg-Str. 1
30625 Hannover

Citak, Mustafa, Dr.
HELIOS ENDO Clinic Hamburg
Holstenstr. 2
22767 Hamburg

Clemens, Ulrich, Dr.
Spitäler fmi ag, Medical Center Frutigen
Adelbodenstr. 27
3714 Frutigen

Dittrich, Stefan, Dr.
Department of Orthopedic Surgery
Gelenk-Zentrum Hietzing
Hietzinger Hauptstr. 34
1130 Vienna

Floerkemeier, Thilo, Dr.
Department of Orthopedic Surgery, Annastift Hospital
Hannover Medical School
Anna-von-Borries-Str. 1–7
30625 Hannover

Franke, Jochen, Dr.
BG Trauma Clinic Ludwigshafen
Ludwig-Guttmann-Str. 13
67071 Ludwigshafen

Gebel, Philipp, MD
University Clinic for Orthopedic Surgery
Bern University Hospital
3010 Bern

Gebhard, Florian, Univ. Prof. Dr.
Department of Orthopedic Trauma
University of Ulm
Steinhövelstr. 9
89075 Ulm

Grützner, Paul Alfred, Prof. Dr.
BG Trauma Clinic Ludwigshafen
Ludwig-Guttmann-Str. 13
67071 Ludwigshafen

Haaker, Rolf, Prof. Dr.
St. Vincenz Hospital
Danziger Str. 17
33034 Brakel

Hawi, Nael, Dr.
Department of Trauma Surgery
Hannover Medical School
Carl-Neuberg-Str. 1
36025 Hannover

Hüfner, Tobias, Prof. Dr.
Department of Trauma Surgery
Hannover Medical School
Carl-Neuberg-Str. 1
36025 Hannover

Imrecke, Julia, Dr.
Department of Trauma Surgery
Hannover Medical School
Carl-Neuberg-Str. 1
30625 Hannover

Ishaque, Bernd, Dr.
Department of Orthopedic Surgery
University Clinic of Giessen and Marburg
Klinikstr. 33
35392 Gießen

Kendoff, Daniel O., PD Dr.
Department of Orthopedic Surgery
ENDO Clinic Hamburg
Holstenstr. 2
22767 Hamburg

Kiefer, Hartmuth, Prof. Dr.
Department of Trauma and Orthopedic Surgery,
Hand and Reconstructive Surgery
LUKAS, Academic Teaching Hospital
Hannover Medical School
Hindenburgstr. 56
32257 Bünde

Konermann, Werner, Prof. Dr.
Kassel Red Cross Hospital
Hansteinstr. 29
34121 Kassel

König, Dietmar Pierre, Prof. Dr.
LVR Clinic for Orthopedics, Viersen
Horionstr. 2
41749 Viersen

Köster, Georg, Prof. Dr.
Specialist Clinic for Orthopedics and Surgery
Waldstr. 13
64653 Lorsch

Krettek, Christian, Prof. Dr.
Department of Trauma Surgery
Hannover Medical School
Carl-Neuberg-Str. 1
30625 Hannover

Lazovic, Djordje, Prof. Dr.
Specialist Clinic for Orthopedics and Orthopedic
Surgery
Pius Hospital
Georgstr. 12
26121 Oldenburg

Lüke, Ulrich
Department of Trauma Surgery
Hannover Medical School
Carl-Neuberg-Str. 1
30625 Hannover

Nöth, Ulrich, Prof.
Orthopedic Center for Musculoskeletal
Research (OZMF)
Institute of Orthopedics
University of Würzburg
Brettreichstr. 11
97074 Würzburg

Ottersbach, Andreas, Dr.
Department of Orthopedics
Oberwallis Hospital Center
Überlandstr. 14
3900 Brig

Ozwald, Markus, Priv.-Doz. Dr.
Department of Trauma and Spinal Surgery
University Hospital Regensburg
Franz-Josef-Strauß-Allee 11
93051 Regensburg

Pearle, Andrew D., Dr.
Department of Orthopedics
Hospital for Special Surgery
72 Street
New York 10021, NY, USA

Radermacher, Klaus, Prof. Dr.-Ing.
Helmholtz Institute for Biomedical Engineering
RWTH Aachen University
Pauwelsstr. 20
52074 Aachen

Richter, Peter, Dr.
Department of Orthopedic Surgery
University of Ulm
Steinhövelstr. 9
89075 Ulm

Riepl, Christoph, Dr.
Department of Orthopedic Surgery
University of Ulm
Steinhövelstr. 9
89075 Ulm

Rudert, Maximilian, Prof. Dr.
Orthopedic Clinic »König Ludwig Haus«,
Institute of Orthopedics
Julius Maximilians University of Würzburg
Brettreichstr. 11
97074 Würzburg

Schnurr, Christoph, PD Dr.
LVR Clinic for Orthopedics, Viersen
Horionstr. 2
41749 Viersen

Scheiderer, Bastian, Dr.
Department of Orthopedic Surgery
University of Ulm
Steinhövelstr. 9
89075 Ulm

Steinert, Andre F., Priv.-Doz. Dr.
Orthopedic Clinic »König Ludwig Haus«,
Institute of Orthopedics
Julius Maximilians University of Würzburg
Brettreichstr. 11
97074 Würzburg

Stübig, Timo, Dr.
Department of Trauma Surgery
Hannover Medical School
Carl-Neuberg-Str. 1
30625 Hannover

Thorey, Fritz, MD, PhD
Center for Hip, Knee and Foot Surgery (HKF)
ATOS Clinic Heidelberg
Bismarckstr. 9-15
69115 Heidelberg

Tibesku, Carsten O., Prof. Dr.
Sporthopaedicum Straubing
Bahnhofplatz 27
94315 Straubing

Windhagen, Henning, Prof. Dr.
Department of Orthopedic Surgery,
Annastift Hospital
Hannover Medical School
Anna-von-Borries-Str. 1–7
30625 Hannover

Introduction

History of Computer-Assisted Surgery

Rolf Haaker

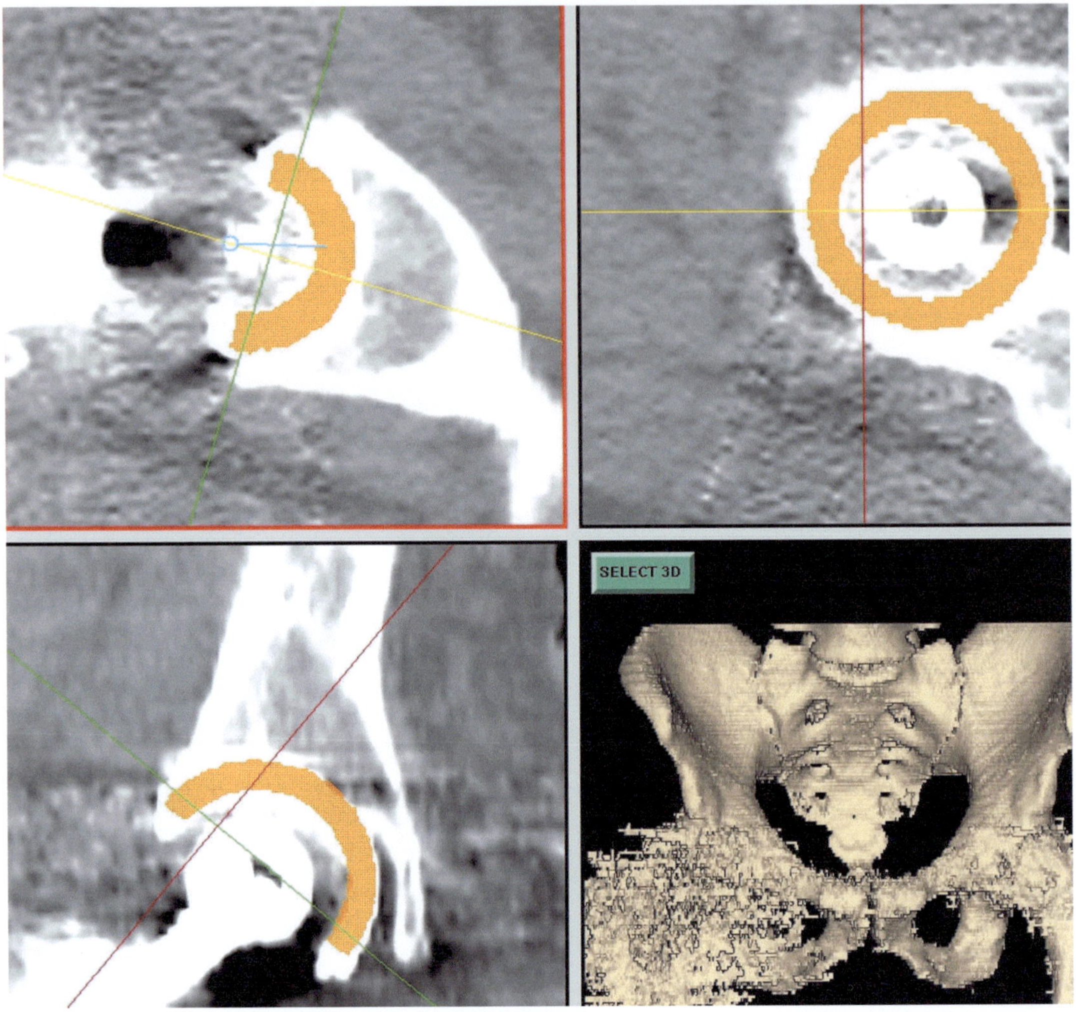

Fig. 1.1 Paired-point matching and virtual cup in a three-dimensional model of the pelvic bone using a CT-based navigation system. A revision case is shown here

When computer-assisted surgery was introduced in the early 1990s, the interest of orthopedic specialists was first focused on robotics. In 1995, when we started with computer navigation for the placement of pedicle screws at Ruhr University Bochum, no-one could imagine that this method would gain entry into orthopedic theaters. It involved time-consuming planning and required preoperative computed tomography (CT); moreover, paired-point and surface matching during the operation was difficult for the surgeon (Fig. 1.1).

Navigation started off with a bad image, because the first problems in robotic surgery had already occurred and enthusiasm for the new computer-based technology was relatively low. Nevertheless, navigation proceeded with CT-based systems (Medivision), and the first software tools dealt with pedicle screw placement and with performing triple osteotomies at the pelvis.

The basis of the scientific technology was the definition of the exact position of any corpus in space according to a coordinate system (called a rigid body). In our first investigations on the biomechanical behavior of multisegmental spinal fusions, we used an ultrasound-based system (Zebris) for movement analysis (Fig. 1.2).

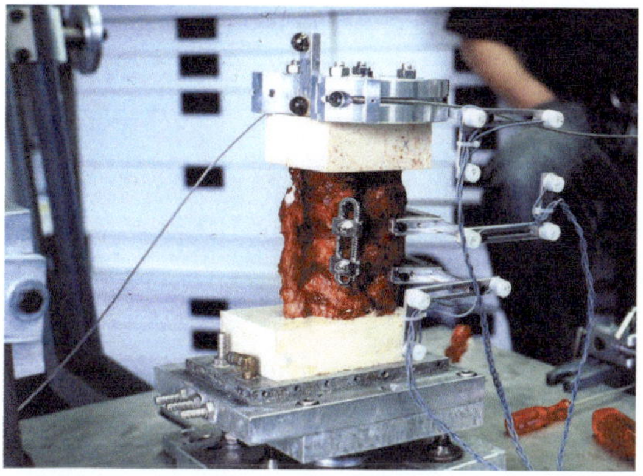

Fig. 1.2 Three-dimensional motion analysis using the Zebris ultrasound motion detector. Motion analysis is shown in a cadaver spine after instrumented fusion

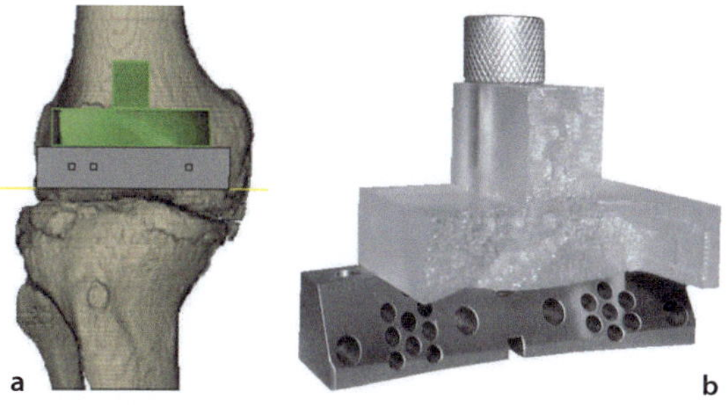

Fig. 1.3a,b Templating with a CAD-formed Plexiglas tool connected to the tibial cutting block of a total knee arthroplasty system. (From Radermacher 2002)

Later, the connection of light-emitting diodes to an infrared camera was used to define the exact position of an object in space. In the future, electromagnetic markers will be used.

Initially, industry did not show much interest in these software tools, because the implants needed for performing a triple osteotomy were relatively cheap and instrumented fusion of the spine was a seldom used procedure. At the same time, Prof. Radermacher in Aachen developed a templating technique particularly for triple osteotomies of the pelvis, but it too was not met with any interest from industry (Fig. 1.3).

The introduction of computer-assisted surgery in total hip and total knee replacement, however, received a lot of attention, even from those in industry.

However, the need to use CT with the first navigation systems so as to gain more precise information and the fact that the surgeon had to deal with the surface and paired-point matching of the case 1 day before the procedure put an end to this type of software. The upcoming technology introduced cinematic-based systems for navigation in total hip arthroplasty (THA) and total knee arthroplasty (TKA) using a database of bones originating from the first years of CT-based navigation systems, which were compared by the computer with the real situation on the operating layer. This set-up drew the attention of a greater collective of surgeons.

Numerous scientific papers in highly cited international journals pointed out the better implant positioning achieved when using navigation systems, but very few papers dealt with the better clinical outcome of patients treated with this technology. This point and the fact that using a navigation system is a time-consuming procedure resulted in the number of navigated TKAs not exceeding 12% of all arthroplasties performed in Germany and 3.6% of all navigated THAs (BQS Study 2005; Haaker et al. 2003, 2005, 2007).

Thus, Bellemans (Leuven, Belgium) pointed out in his paper »Navigation and CAS. Is D-Day Approaching?«: »Where are the papers that demonstrate better clinical performance or better survivorship for cases operated on with navigation? Where are the clinical data that confirm that improved accuracy as obtained with navigation leads to better clinical results?« (Bellemans 2009).

On the one hand, navigation answered many open questions concerning the range of motion in THA, which in the last few years led to ceramic heads with greater diameters to prevent subluxation or impingement to the inlays. The position of the acetabular component itself does not seem to be that important, because placement in the so-called safe zone of Lewinnek was not always sufficient. On the other hand, the allegedly badly positioned cups did not always dislocate during the first months or show increased wear of the polyethylene inlays. Questions on the reconstruction of leg length and offset were increasingly raised and thus the combined anteversion of the stem and acetabular component became

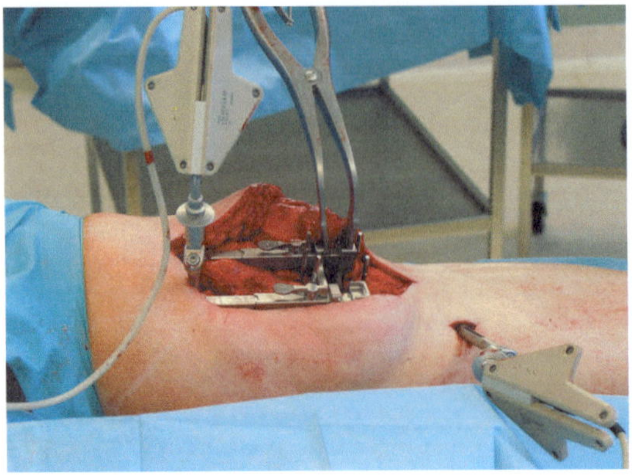

■ **Fig. 1.4** Soft tissue balancing in second-generation navigation systems. The OrthoPilot® 4.0 software is shown here

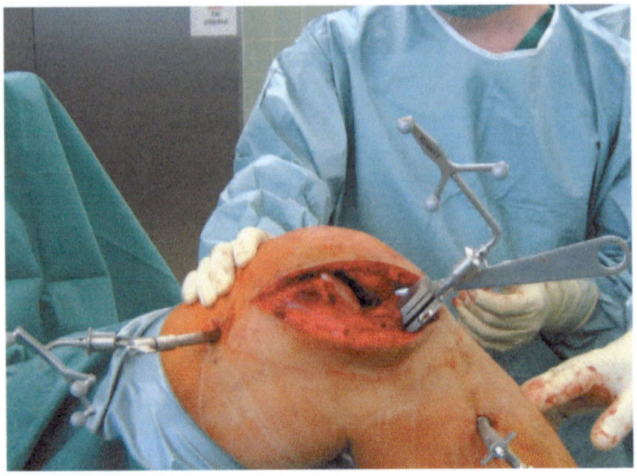

■ **Fig. 1.5** Navigation of the tibial cutting block in a Uniglide® UKA

the focus of surgeons who perform the »femur-first technique« in THAs.

In TKAs, malrotation of the femoral component and its consequences for anterior knee pain was a hot topic for surgeons, including the question of reconstruction within the Mikulicz line.

In the evolution of navigation systems, several companies such as Brainlab, Medtronic, Braun-Aesculap (OrthoPilot®), and others developed software that addressed soft tissue balancing in TKA as well as rotational aspects of the femoral component (■ Fig. 1.4). The unsolved problem was the definition of rotation of the tibial component. Nearly all of the second-generation navigation systems facilitated soft tissue balancing.

Special software tools were developed for unicompartmental knee arthroplasty (UKA), shoulder joint replacement, and intervertebral disc prostheses. Nevertheless, most surgeons did not use navigation systems because of the high time consumption in the operating theater, the difficult software, and the complicated workflow.

Against this backdrop, industry made a final attempt to create more user-friendly navigation systems resulting in the introduction of iPod® navigation by Brainlab.

Several problems in joint replacement were addressed and solved with the help of navigation systems, such as range of motion in THA, or malrotation of the femoral components in TKA, or the slope in UKA. The author, with the support of CAS Erlangen/Siemens, developed a navigation system to be used with the Uniglide® UKA system (■ Fig. 1.5) (Haaker et al. 2007).

A renaissance in templating technology was witnessed in 2009, especially in TKAs. The producer ConforMIS (known for its CAD-shaped knee spacers) developed, under the leadership of Fritz and coworkers, a new technique to create special templates for UKAs and bicompartmental knee arthroplasties based on the data of a CT scan of the knee and a single-leg stance x-ray. In these special cases, a custom-made prosthesis was created fitting the individual patient. The technology did not differ so much from the first attempts described by Radermacher et al., but surprisingly less criticism about the use of CT was expressed at this time (■ Fig. 1.6).

Shortly afterward, other manufacturers such as Smith & Nephews (Visionaire), Zimmer (PSI), and Depuy (Tru-Match) developed a templating system based on CT or magnetic resonance imaging (MRI) data to create single-use cutting blocks for creating serial knee prostheses. Companies such as Medacta (My Knee) and Symbios (Knee-Plan) from Switzerland also developed this new technology.

Bellemans's comment that 2011 was the D-Day for navigation was made because today, 10 years after the introduction of this system, there are only a few papers on the clinical outcome of navigated TKAs. Nevertheless, these reports raised interest in the even better clinical outcomes 10 years after computer-navigated TKA in comparison to conven-

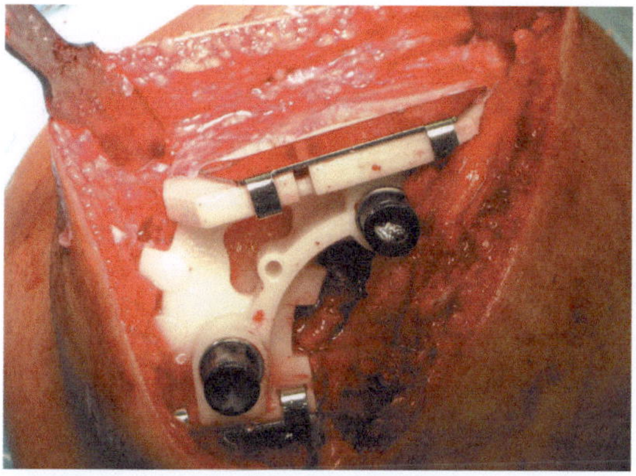

■ **Fig. 1.6** A ConforMIS iDuo individual femoral cutting block connected to the femoral bone

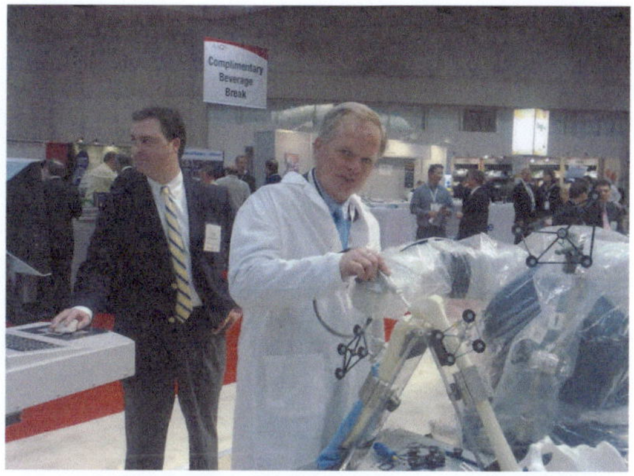

■ **Fig. 1.7** A Mako System robotic arm at the 2011 AAOS meeting in San Diego

tional TKAs. Thus, Baumbach (Baumbach 2012) showed a revision rate of 23% in conventional TKA compared to 5.6% after navigated cases using the same implant (Search Evolution; B. Braun, Aesculap). The revision for both the TKA and the conventionally navigated cases was due to the varus that was seen within the 10 years after the procedure; however, the varus for the navigated cases was a median of 0.4°–2.9° and for the conventional cases a median of 3.2°–5.6°. Thus, the conclusion that exact implant positioning increases the longevity of implants could be drawn for the first time. However, there seems to be a special interest in computer-assisted tools to position implants more precisely than in conventionally handled cases.

Thus, even the robotic systems that »died« in the first few years of the twenty-first century are now taking on a new role in UKA (Mako Systems) and THA (■ Fig. 1.7). Numerous medical engineers are working on the development of new, simple navigation systems using electromagnetic markers, load force analysis, and other tools.

In my opinion, the chapter on robotic systems that opened in the early 1990s will not be closed before attractive technologies are available for performing TKAs within the Mikulicz line and with an exact slope of the tibial component under the best-balanced ligament tension using a small computerized device. Especially in the United States, where operating theater time is paid by the minute, the technology should not waste any time at all. This is basically why templating systems were developed, because they allow engineers to deal with a case long before it goes to the operating theater. Even the cost-saving production of single-use cutting blocks is of interest to industry. But is the surgeon really interested in a situation where an engineer decides on the best rotation of femoral and tibial components in TKA? I cannot imagine that this is the final solution. Particularly in countries with diagnosis-related group payments (DRGs), this type of TKA is too costly to perform and the preoperative x-ray load is too high (Ottersbach and Haaker 2005; Victor et al. 2009).

Navigation based on 3D fluoroscopy, which was introduced in the 1990s, is a helpful tool in trauma surgery but also in orthopedic surgery. 3D fluoroscopy is useful for judging pedicle screw placement after instrumented spinal fusion as well as rotational aspects of femoral components in TKAs (Beck et al. 2009). Additional features of this method are presented in Chaps. 17 and 18 of this book (■ Fig. 1.8).

Thus, we have to wait and see how the development of new technologies advances. I believe we now have enough experience on hand with the available technologies for the interested readers to form their own opinion about this popular subspecialty of orthopedic surgery.

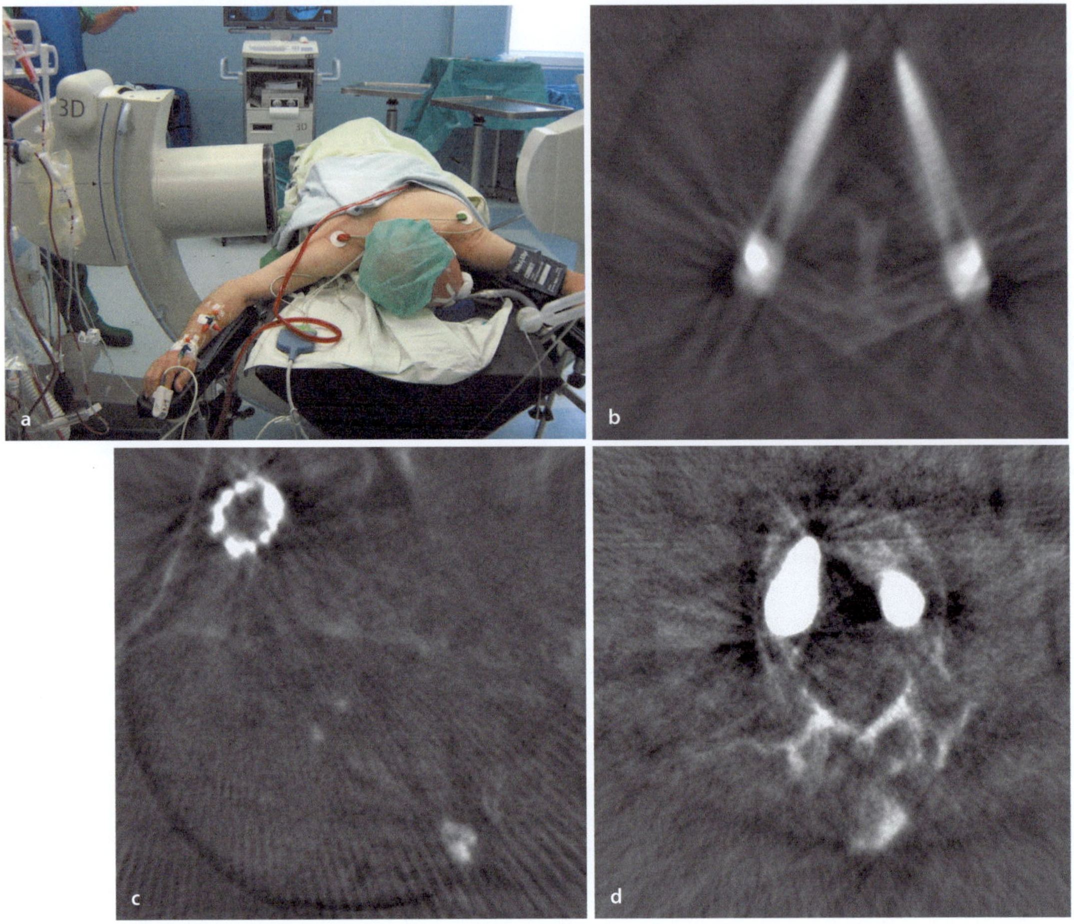

Fig. 1.8 **a** The Arcadis Orbic 3D fluoroscope after an instrumented spinal fusion. **b** Pedicle screws on a 3D fluoroscopy scan. **c** Distraction cage in the sacroiliac joint on a 3D scan. **d** Kyphoplasty on a 3D scan

References

Baumbach JA (2012) 10-Jahres-Ergebnisse hinsichtlich Lockerungsrate navigierter versus nicht navigierter Knietotalendoprothesen Typ Aesculap Search aus dem Jahr 1999 Inaugural-Dissertation Ruhr Universität Bochum; vorab publiziert. Int. CAOS-meeting Seoul 2012

Beck M, Moritz K, Gierer P, Gradl G, Harms C, Mittlmeier T (2009) Intraoperative control of pedicle screws using 3-d fluoroscopy. A prospective study in the treatment of thorakolumbar fractures. Z Orthop 147:37–42

Bellemans J (2009) Navigation and CAS: is D-Day approaching? Knee Surg Sports Arthrosc 17:1141–1142

Haaker RG, Stockheim M, Kamp M, Proff G, Breitenfelder J, Ottersbach A (2005) Computer-assisted navigation increases precision of component placement in total knee arthroplasty. Clin Orthop 433 152–159

Haaker RG, Tiedjen K, Ottersbach A, Rubenthaler F, Stockheim M, Stiehl JB (2007) Comparison of conventional versus computer – navigated acetabular component insertion. J Arthroplasty 22:151–160

Haaker RG, Tiedjen K, Rubenthaler F, Stockheim M (2003) Computerassistierte Hüftpfannennavigation bei primär und sekundär dysplastischen Ausgangssituationen. Z Orthop 141:105–112

Haaker R, Wojciechowski M, Patzer P, Willburger RE, Senkal M, Engelhardt M (2007) Minimally invasive unicondylar knee replacement with computer navigation. Orthopaede 35:1073–1080

Ottersbach A, Haaker R (2005) Optimization of cup positioning in THA – comparison between conventional mechanical instrumentation and computer-assisted implanted cups by using the Orthopilot navigation system. Z Orthop 143:611–615

Portheine F, Ohnsorge J, Schkommodau E, Radermacher K (2002) CT-basierte Planung und DISOS-Schablonennavigation in der Kniegelenkendoprothetik. In: Konermann W, Haaker R (eds) Navigation und Robotik in der Gelenk- und Wirbelsäulenchirurgie. Springer, Berlin Heidelberg New York, pp 262–272

Victor J, Van Doninck D, Labey L, Innocenti B, Parizel PM, Bellemans (2009) How precise can bony landmarks be determined on a CT scan of the knee? Knee 16:358–365

Renaissance of Computer-Assisted Orthopedic Surgery with Individual Templates: Evolution or Revolution?

Klaus Radermacher

The principle of individual templates was originally introduced and developed by our team at the Helmholtz Institute for Biomedical Engineering, RWTH Aachen University of Technology, Aachen, Germany, in the early 1990s. This contribution provides a summary of these early developments and experiences in the field of computer-assisted orthopedic surgery. It includes an analysis of major key factors of the general acceptance of this approach in today's clinical practice. The conclusion points out specific aspects of earlier developments that could still be considered for an optimization of current commercial implementations, and it emphasizes the limitations of the individual template approach justifying the need for additional complementary tools such as navigation and robotics in computer-assisted orthopedic surgery – depending on the specific clinical needs and applications.

2.1 Historical Background and Evolution

Shortly after the introduction of three-dimensional computed tomography (3D-CT) imaging with the related image-processing and 3D reconstruction techniques, the manufacturing of customized physical models of the patient's anatomy was proposed in the early 1980s for surgical planning as well as for custom implants in total hip replacement or bone tumor surgery. However, these approaches closed only part of the loop between 3D medical image acquisition and personalized surgical therapy. At the same time, in industrial applications, robotic systems were established linking a programmed computer-based plan of a 3D trajectory or positioning of 3D (e.g., computer manufactured) objects in a defined reference coordinate system within the manufacturing process. Consequently, following the general principles of stereotactic interventions, the first robotic systems were proposed for stereotactic neurosurgery and later for other medical applications, too, such as radiation therapy and orthopedics by Hap Paul and Russ Taylor in 1989. The first robotic implementation of total hip arthroplasty (THA) took place in human subjects in 1991 (Taylor et al. 1996). Surgical navigation technology was introduced by Adams and coworkers in the late 1980s (Adams et al. 1990) using the same basic technology as for 3D reconstruction and registration, but enabling visual feedback of an anatomical location even on non-planned trajectories of manually handled instruments localized by mechanical coordinate measuring arms. Mechanical localizers were later replaced by ultrasound-based and then optical (as well as electromagnetic) tracking systems. The principle of navigation for orthopedic surgery was introduced by Nolte et al. (1995).

The fundamental requirement for the positioning of screws, cuts, and implant devices in orthopedic surgery is to realize a static position in the patient's anatomical coordinate system according to a defined, preferably computer-based plan. In industrial environments (for carpenters, metal workers, and designers), the standard solution for this problem is to manufacture a specific template or jig system enabling repeatable manual positioning with high accuracy and constraining the tool or device to be positioned to the defined location.

In 1988, Prof. Wessinghage (Bad Abbach, Germany), a friend of my father's, asked me whether there could be a better *standardization* of the large instrument sets used in total knee arthroplasty that generated high costs and logistical problems in clinical routine. However, the main problem of the large instrument sets and jig systems for cutting and drilling the implant seat for knee endoprostheses was the missing link between the implant geometry (implicitly included in the implant-specific cutting blocks) on the one hand and the patients' anatomy and surgical plan on the other hand. Therefore, many components were necessary for measurements and trials during surgery. Taking into account the state of the art of 3D imaging and reconstruction, I proposed to go the opposite way of standardization, by applying state-of-the-art computer-integrated planning and numerically controlled (NC) manufacturing technology to provide CT-based personalized instrumentation for each patient using all-in-one cutting blocks for the tibial and femoral bone preparation. Being an undergraduate mechanical engineering student, the feedback I received from experienced engineers was that this would have many technical hurdles and be a far-too-expensive, crazy idea …!

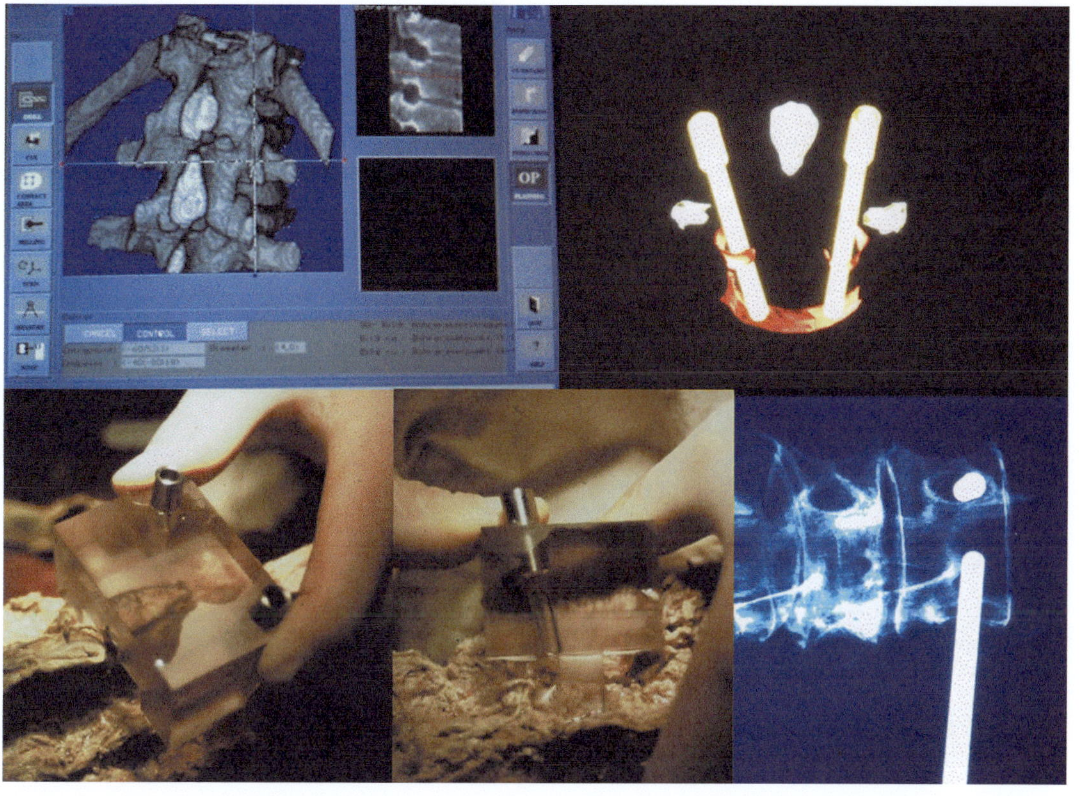

Fig. 2.1 Early cadaver feasibility study on pedicle screw placement with individual templates: CT-based planning (*upper left*), resulting plan including planned bores, critical bone surfaces (pedicles and anterior vertebral bone layer), as well as contact areas for the custom jig (*upper right*). Cadaver laboratory: checking fit by haptics and visually (note the effect of transparent wet jigs; *lower left and center*); x-ray check with inserted rod (*lower right*)

In 1991, as a young PhD student at the Helmholtz Institute for Biomedical Engineering in Aachen, I had the opportunity to reexplore my idea. I was invited by Prof. H.-W. Staudte, head of the department for orthopedic surgery and traumatology at the district hospital Marienhoehe in Würselen, Germany, to visit a scoliosis intervention. He asked me whether we could develop technical means to support the placement of pedicle screws, which could be easily applied and handled during surgery, in these pathological situations of high interindividual variability.

We acquired a CT image dataset of a macerated dry lumbar spine specimen, transferred it via 8« floppy disc (3–4 CT slices per disc!) to a PDP11 and via Kermit (9600 Baud) to a standard PC. Segmentation of bone contours was done after standard thresholding and contour stacks were transferred via Kermit serial data transfer interface software and on the basis of a custom GPL script to an ICEM DDN CAD/CAM workstation (Control Data Inc.). The initial design of an individual template consisted in a basic jig block with four contact areas on the bilateral transverse processes and lamina arcs. Two bores were defined in the center of the pedicles going through the jig block (later on equipped with metal sleeves). The area of the contact surfaces was manually reconstructed by interpolation using standard CAD features. NC-milling paths were generated using the ICEM DDN interfaces, postprocessed, and sent to a three-axis MAHO milling machine. After manufacturing, the template was manually positioned for the first time on the bone specimen and showed an excellent fit and repositioning accuracy of the pedicle bores. Further trials were conducted with fresh cadaver material, and

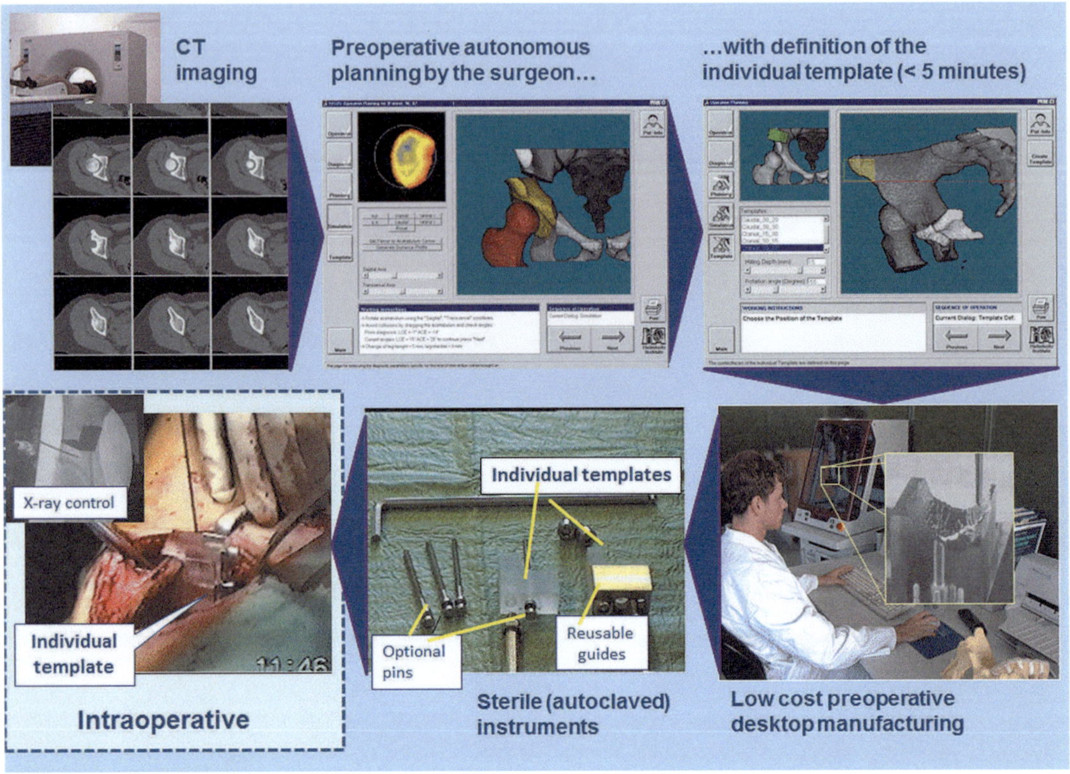

Fig. 2.2 DISOS desktop image processing, surgical planning, and manufacturing of custom jigs for a periacetabular repositioning osteotomy

bores in both pedicles were checked with an x-ray image (Fig. 2.1) (Radermacher et al. 1993a, 1993b, 1994a, 1994b, 1995, 1996a, 1996b, 1998, 1999; Rau et al. 1995; Staudte et al. 1998). Encouraged by the results of this feasibility study, a patent application on the principle of individual templates was filed in 1992 (German Patent DE 4219939; International Patent Application WO 1993/025157). We offered this patent to different companies – to Smith & Nephew as well as to Aesculap, 1993–1995 – who were not interested at that time because of some technical hurdles and the questionable commercial applicability. Owing to the high cost of international patenting, we were only able to continue with the German patent, which finally expired in June 2012.

After these initial proof-of-concept studies, we focused on the development of an integrated *d*esktop *i*mage processing and planning *s*ystem for *o*rthopedic *s*urgery (DISOS). Moreover, we analyzed further clinical applications. In this context, Prof. Staudte proposed the periacetabular triple osteotomy according to Tönnis as another application that needed image-based 3D planning and intraoperative support. Major hurdles in this procedure are the low case numbers leading to limited learning curves for the surgeons as well as the high 3D complexity of the osteotomies and the repositioning of the acetabular fragment. Consequently, the first clinical application of individual templates supporting a periacetabular triple osteotomy was successfully tested in 1993 (Radermacher et al. 1994a, 1994b, 1995, 1996a, 1996b, 1999; Portheine et al. 1996). In the following years, we developed a DISOS planning module enabling the surgeon to plan the osteotomy intervention within 5–10 min after receiving the CT dataset using a standard desktop PC. We used desktop NC-milling technology (a three-axis milling system for about € 5,000) adapted to the planning system. The surgeon was able to automatically manufacture and sterilize the

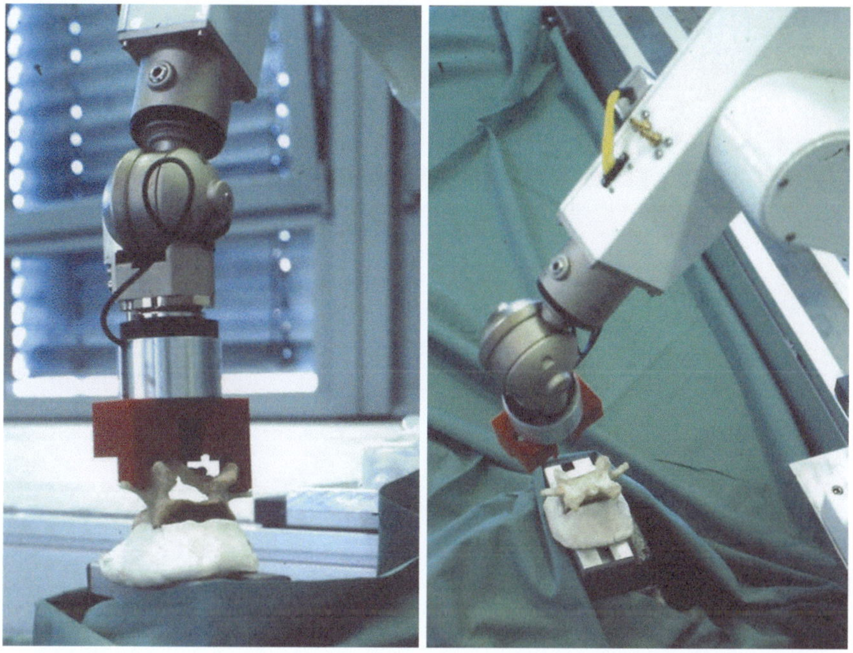

Fig. 2.3 First concept study on robot registration with an individual template (for pedicle screw insertion) during 1993–1995. Template-based manual registration of a PUMA 260 robot (*left*) and planning-based indication of the pedicle axis using a robot-based laser pointer (*right*)

polycarbonate template within 60 min after electronic transfer of the CT dataset (Fig. 2.2) (Portheine et al. 1997, 1998; Radermacher 1999; Radermacher et al. 1999, 1996b). (Of note, today standard processing times for custom jigs of commercial providers using remote image processing, planning, and generative manufacturing techniques are up to 6 weeks and longer!)

A subsequent series of 54 triple pelvic acetabular osteotomies (conventional vs. template based) demonstrated the short-term clinical benefit of the template-based procedure, while no significant long-term differences between the two procedures were found (Staudte et al. 1997, 1998, 2002, 2003; Radermacher et al. 1998; Radermacher 1999; Schiffers et al. 2000; Schkommodau et al. 2001).

The system is commercially available with the OrthoTAIX planning unit (SurgiTAIX AG, Aachen, Germany). Further studies on spinal applications included a cadaver study on different design approaches (Schkommodau et al. 2001, 2002, 2003; Birnbaum et al. 2001). Moreover, a comparative clinical study using a Sofamor Danek Stealth Station Navigation System vs. individual templates showed that there were no differences in accuracy; however, the template technology offered significantly shorter intraoperative set-up and operating times (Schkommodau et al. 2000).

Furthermore, we demonstrated the use of an individual template for the registration of a robot-based laser pointer for positioning and orienting pedicle screws in a laboratory study. We showed that there was a very simple and intuitive registration of the robot with an individual template and the subsequent planning-based positioning of the laser by the robot device (PUMA 260, Stäubli) (Fig. 2.3) (Radermacher et al. 1996b).

The first clinical study on individual templates for total knee replacement surgery using an integrated preoperative desktop planning and manufacturing system and intraoperative custom jigs in ten cases was conducted in 2000/2001 (Portheine et al. 2001; Portheine 2004). The resulting alignments were all within a 3° boundary and the cut–suture time in these first ten trials was 35–70 min (Portheine et al. 2001). We encountered several technical

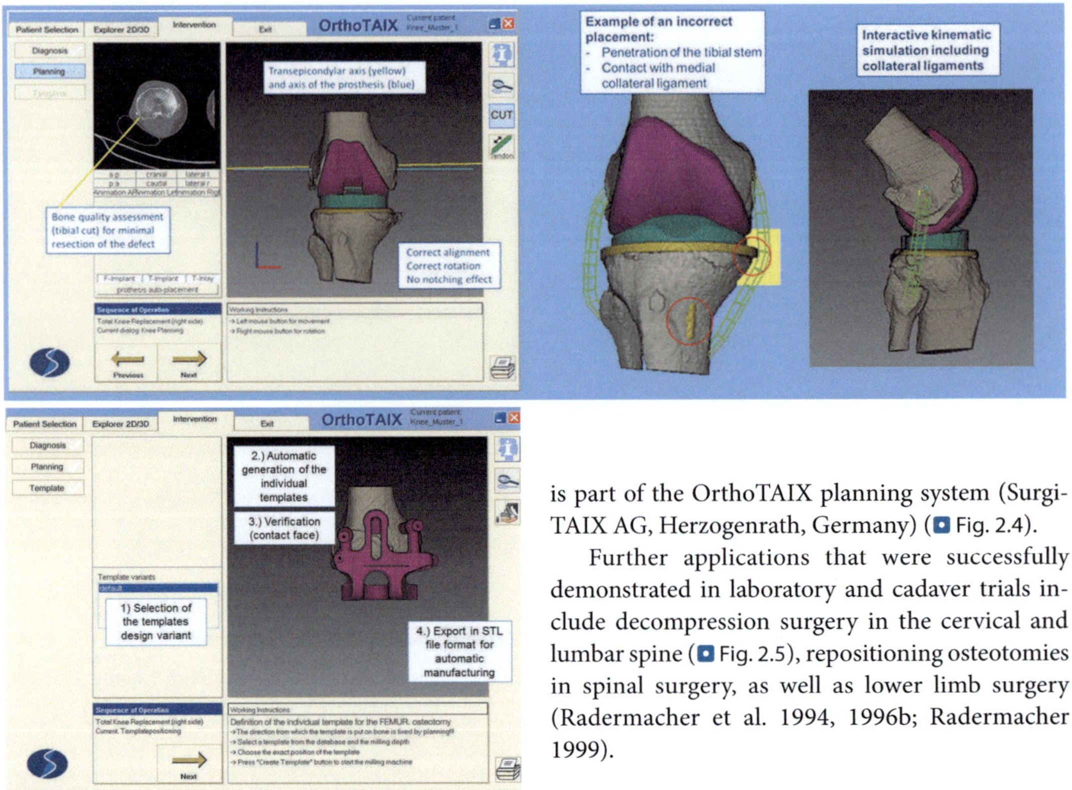

Fig. 2.4a,b Example of the OrthoTAIX Planning system (SurgiTAIX AG, Aachen, Germany) for the planning and manufacturing of custom jigs for total knee replacement surgery. Implant planning (**a**) and definition of the custom jig (**b**)

challenges at that time. For example, we were not able to reach an agreement with major implant manufacturers in order to have the CAD implant geometry data of the state-of-the-art endoprostheses. Thus, the implant geometry was not properly defined. As a result, 3D planning was not very efficient and lacked accuracy. A multicut cutting block for the femoral component, as is offered by some manufacturers today, was not possible based on the available 3D CAD implant geometry data. In view of some of these challenges and the technical capabilities available at the time, further development of this application for clinical routine use was not possible at that time. Moreover, many orthopedic surgeons felt that there was no relevant clinical application of custom templates to knee replacement surgery. Today, our desktop planning module is part of the OrthoTAIX planning system (SurgiTAIX AG, Herzogenrath, Germany) (Fig. 2.4).

Further applications that were successfully demonstrated in laboratory and cadaver trials include decompression surgery in the cervical and lumbar spine (Fig. 2.5), repositioning osteotomies in spinal surgery, as well as lower limb surgery (Radermacher et al. 1994, 1996b; Radermacher 1999).

Clinical and laboratory applications of individual template technology: 1993–2000 (see References)

- Spine surgery
  - Pedicle screw placement (clinical study)
  - Dorsal Hirayabashi open-door decompression (cadaver study)
  - Ventral decompression (cadaver study)
  - Ventral repositioning osteotomies (laboratory study)
- Hip surgery
  - Total hip surgery (laboratory concept study)
  - Intertrochanteric osteotomy (including punction of bone cyst; lab study)
  - Periacetabular repositioning osteotomy (Tönnis; clinical study)
  - Spherical periacetabular osteotomy (laboratory study and first cadaver study)
- Knee surgery
  - Total knee arthroplasty (clinical study)

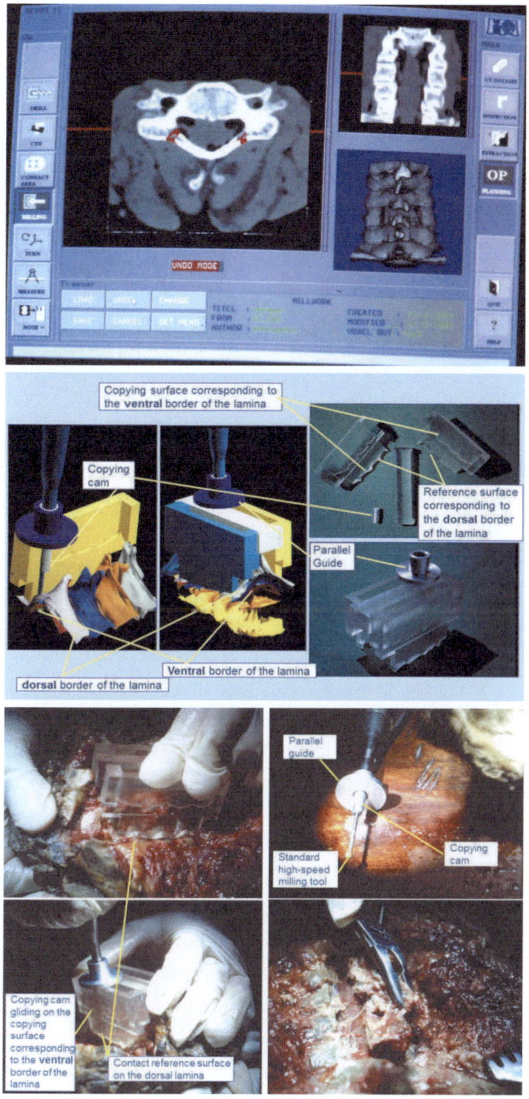

Fig. 2.5a–c Open-door decompression in the cervical spine. CT-based planning with DISOS (**a**): CAD-based design of contact faces and copying surfaces guiding the milling tool equipped with a copying camera to limit the cutting depth to the frontal surface of the lamina (**b**). (**c**): Cadaver test showing the efficient preservation of a bony hinge on one side and of the dura on the contralateral side

2.2 From Concept to Broad Clinical Acceptance: Evolution or Revolution?

Our early work on individual templates in orthopedic surgery has clearly laid the foundation for the entire field of patient-specific instruments that is expanding so rapidly now. Many clinically important and meaningful enhancements of our concept have been made in the intervening years. Today, some modern jig designs utilize the shape information of the damaged or normal cartilage portions, thereby improving the accuracy of intraoperative registration. In addition, by including the shape information of combinations of articular cartilage or subchondral bone and cortical bone, the intraoperative registration accuracy of the jigs can be further improved. Modern jigs also use the condylar shape and geometry for the distal femur including the cartilage for accurately referencing the jig during surgery. Similarly, on the tibial side, modern jigs now also reference the articular surface of the medial and/or lateral tibial plateau as well as other tibial plateau structures such as the tibial spines, while our early concept templates were designed to position purely on anterior bone, avoiding these areas.

2.2.1 Breakthroughs Toward Modern Patient-Specific Instruments

What have been the key elements for the renaissance and breakthrough of the individual template approach in recent years?

- Firstly, computer-assisted orthopedic surgery (CAOS) technology such as image- and planning-guided robotics as well as navigation created new clinical pathways that had not been sufficiently advanced, established, or accepted before (e.g., CT or MRI processing, derivation of articular shapes including cartilage, registration, 3D planning, and computer-assisted surgery).
- Secondly, CAOS technology allowed for more research and discussion because it offered the possibility to systematically analyze and quantify surgical errors and deviations from

the optimal outcome. This in turn made surgeons aware of the deficiencies of conventional techniques and of the options for technical support.

- The initial technical appeal and enthusiasm regarding navigation and robot-assisted surgery – in contrast to a simple piece of plastic (a custom jig), the somewhat »magic« connection of the cursor showing the tip of the navigated instrument on the image data display or even the robot moving the instrument certainly had a better appeal and fascination – today is replaced by the pragmatism of demanding technical support with higher efficiency especially regarding operating time and costs.
- The availability and quality of volumetric imaging (spatial resolution, fidelity of image data, true volumetric data with volumetric acquisition) such as CT and MRI increased and the radiation exposure associated with a standard CT of the spine, hip, or knee decreased significantly.
- The pathways, speed, and routine use of data transfer via intranets and the Internet have been established and their routine use has been broadly accepted in the medical community too. Moreover, the generation of surgeons has changed and today surgeons use a computer as a standard tool for their daily work.
- The structure in hospitals has also changed and people are accepting 6 weeks between a CT scan and an operation, which would have been unacceptable 10–20 years ago.

The availability and broad industrial application of enhanced rapid prototyping (generative) manufacturing technology such as selective laser sintering and melting technology together with biocompatible polymers have enabled the mass manufacturing of custom devices by service providers. By contrast, our comparative studies in the early 1990s using early stereolithography vs. low-cost NC-milling machines showed (bearing in mind that no biocompatible photopolymer was available at that time) that the time for manufacturing of a typical custom jig with a milling machine could be 10–15 min (based on semifinished products) vs. 1–2 days using a rapid prototyping machine. The costs per jig are comparable or even lower with milling.

Today, custom jigs are used in dental implantology, craniofacial surgery, repositioning osteotomies of the upper and lower extremities, and hip and knee surgery. Some of the current implementations and applications of different providers are presented in this book.

2.3 Conclusion and Outlook

Although important technical advances have been achieved, some major features have still not been implemented by most providers of custom jigs today. The (re-)implementation of some of these features could be one objective of further developments:

- In 1994/1995, our DISOS process for the planning and manufacturing of individual templates provided a planning system for a surgeon's standard desktop PC and enabled the surgeon to use an autoclaved custom jig within 60 min after receiving the CT data (◘ Fig. 2.2). Today, for some manufacturers, the planning is done by technicians in Malaysia (hopefully checked and confirmed by the surgeon) and provided 6 weeks after the submission of the CT or MR dataset. The use of MR data is potentially prone to errors due to spatial distortion and should be checked carefully on a case-by-case basis.
- Since 1993, we have been using transparent material (polycarbonate) for the custom jigs, as this enables an easy visual check of the fit of the contact face on bone (see ◘ Fig. 2.1): a wet surface of the template together with a direct contact on the bone enables a clear view on the bone surface.
- In 1998, we introduced a mathematical approach for constraint analysis of the template fit on bone avoiding uncertain positioning during operation (Radermacher et al. 2000b; Radermacher 1999). The method showed a high sensitivity and predictability for uncertain contact areas defined during the planning process. More complex designs of custom jigs also enabling the guidance of 2D and 3D milling tasks have been proposed and evaluated in

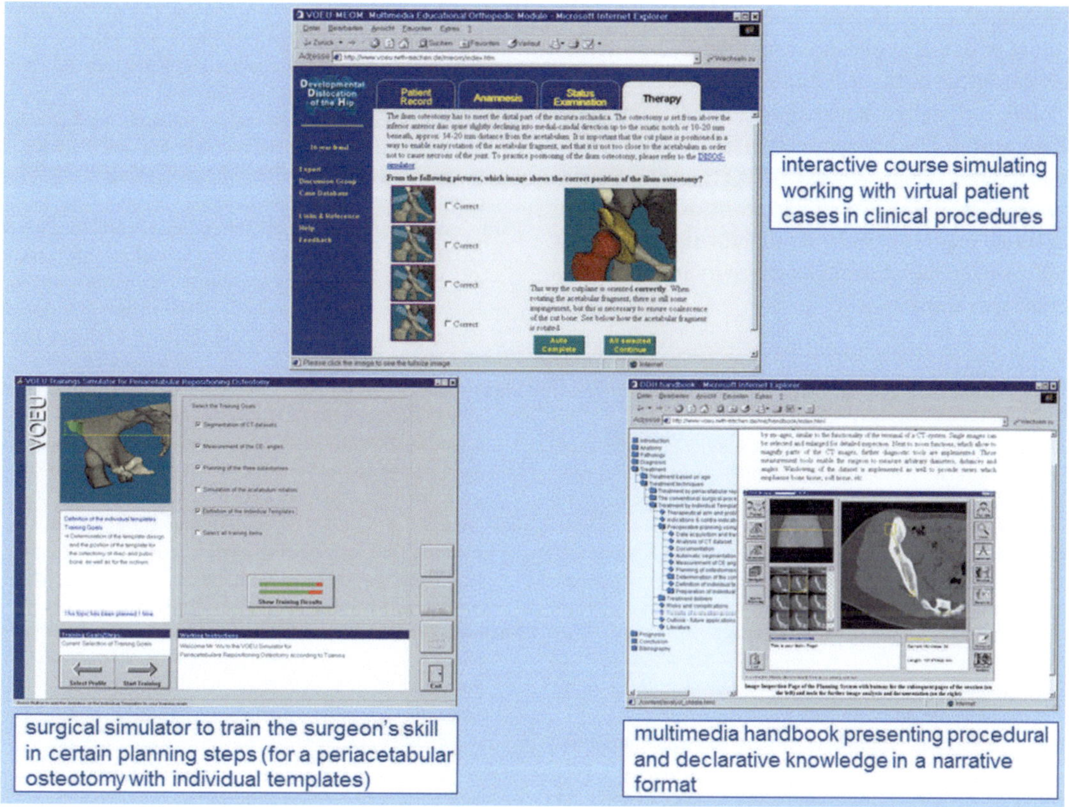

Fig. 2.6 VOEU surgical training environment for education and training in custom jig technology

our early work but have still not been adopted by most providers today (Radermacher et al. 1994a; Radermacher 1999).

- The use of individual templates for an easy and fast intraoperative registration of navigation or robot systems (see Fig. 2.3) could be further explored.
- In the framework of the EU-Project VOEU (Virtual Orthopaedic European University), an Internet-based platform for education and training of CAOS technology has been implemented including specific modules (Fig. 2.6), e.g., for periacetabular osteotomies with custom jigs (Radermacher et al. 2001).

In conclusion, individual templates (custom jigs) today are an accepted solution especially in knee surgery and potentially useful for many other applications. However, they will not replace navigation, smart instruments, or synergistic robotics for many other applications in traumatology and orthopedic surgery.

We look forward to seeing some of our current research in these domains (www.meditec.hia.rwth-aachen.de) achieving the same success as the custom jig approach we proposed more than 20 years ago. However, one lesson learned from previous developments in computer-assisted surgery certainly is that a critical analysis of the available technical possibilities vs. the clinical needs and surgical reality in daily clinical routine is always recommendable. This is one reason why it took more than 20 years from concept to broad clinical implementation of this technology in knee replacement surgery.

2.4 Acknowledgments

Special thanks to Prof. Hans-Walter Staudte, MD, who was the first clinical promoter and user of the individual template technique. His vision of additional potential applications and his interest in the development of the technique have been crucial. I would especially like to thank Frank Portheine, PhD, and Erik Schkommodau, PhD, who provided outstanding major contributions regarding the development and implementation of our integrated desktop planning and manufacturing system for individual templates and its experimental as well as clinical evaluation.

References

Adams L, Krybus W, Meyer-Ebrecht D, Rueger R, Gilsbach JM, Moesges R, Schloendorff G (1990) Computer assisted surgery. IEEE Computer Graphics and Applications 10: 43–51

Birnbaum K, Schkommodau E, Decker N, Prescher A, Klapper U, Radermacher K (2001) Computer assisted orthopedic surgery with individual templates and comparison to conventional methods. Spine 26:365–369

Nolte LP, Visarius H, Arm E, Langlotz F, Schwarzenbach O, Zamorano L (1995) Computer aided fixation of spinal implants. J Image Guid Surg 1:88–93

Portheine F (2004) Modellbasierte Operationsplanung in der Orthopädischen Chirurgie. Shaker Verlag, Aachen

Portheine F, Zimolong A, Radermacher K, Rau G (1996) Präoperative Planung und Planungsumsetzung in der computerunterstützten orthopädischen Chirurgie. In: Lehmann T, Scholl I, Spitzer K (eds) Bildverarbeitung für die Medizin. Proceedings zum Aachener Workshop, 8–9 November 1996, Verlag der Augustinus Buchhandlung Aachen, pp 185–190

Portheine F, Radermacher K, Zimolong A, Anton M, Eichhorn C, Staudte H-W, Rau G (1997) Development of a clinical demonstrator for computer assisted orthopedic surgery with CT-image based individual templates. In: Lemke et al (eds) Computer assisted radiology and surgery. Elsevier, Amsterdam, pp 944–949

Portheine F, Zimolong A, Radermacher K, Rau G (1998) Entwicklung eines klinischen Demonstrators für die computerunterstützte Orthopädische Chirurgie mit CT-bildbasierten Individualschablonen. In: Lehmann T, Metzler V, Spitzer K, Tolxdorff T (eds) Bildverarbeitung für die Medizin 1998. Springer, Berlin Heidelberg New York pp 149–153

Portheine F, Radermacher K, Staudte H-W (2000a) Potentiale der CT-basierten Planung und schablonengestützten Ausführung in der Hüft- und Kniechirurgie. Orthopädische Praxis, 36:786–791

Portheine F, Radermacher K, Staudte H-W, Rau G (2000b) Computerunterstützte CT-bildbasierte Operationsplanung bei Umstellungsosteotomien. Zeitschrift für Biomedizinische Technik 45:202–203

Portheine F, Frömel M, Radermacher K (2001) Computerunterstützte Knie-Totalendoprothetik mit planungsspezifischen Bearbeitungsschablonen. Zeitschrift für Biomedizinische Technik 46:370–371

Portheine F, Ohnsorge JAK, Frömel M, Radermacher K (2002a) Modellierung von Bandstrukturen bei der CT-bildbasierten Planung knieendoprothetischer Eingriffe. Biomedizinische Technik 47:53–56

Portheine F, Ohnsorge J, Schkommodau E, Radermacher K (2002b) CT- basierte Planung und Schablonennavigation für die Kniegelenk-Endoprothetik. In: Konermann W, Haaker R (eds) Navigation und Robotik in der Gelenk- und Wirbelsäulenchirurgie. Springer, Berlin Heidelberg New York, pp 262–269

Portheine F, Ohnsorge JAK, Schkommodau E, Radermacher K (2003) CT-based planning and individual template navigation in TKA. In: Stiehl JB, Konermann WH, Haaker RG (eds) Navigation and robotics in total joint and spine surgery. Springer, Berlin Heidelberg New York, pp 336-342

Radermacher K (1999) Computerunterstützte Operationsplanung und -ausführung mittels individueller Bearbeitungsschablonen in der Orthopädie. Dissertation, RWTH Aachen

Radermacher K (2002) MRCAS in Forschung und/oder breiter klinischer Anwendung – Rechtfertigung, Alternativen und Perspektiven. In: Labs K, Zippel H (eds) Stand und Perspektiven der computer-assistierten Chirurgie. Uni-Med-Verlag, Bremen, pp 145–152

Radermacher K, Rau G (2000) Computerassistierte Planung und Operation in der Orthopädie. Orthopädische Praxis 36:731–737

Radermacher K, Staudte H-W, Rau G (1993a) Computer assisted matching of planning and execution in orthopedic surgery. In: Proceedings of the IEEE EMBS, San Diego, 1993, pp 946–947

Radermacher K, Rau G., Staudte HW (1993b) Computer integrated advanced orthopedics. In: Proceedings of the 2nd European Conference in Engineering and Medicine, Stuttgart, 1993, pp 1–2

Radermacher K, Staudte H-W, Rau G (1994a) Computer assisted orthopaedic surgery by means of individual templates – aspects and analysis of potential applications. In: DiGioia III A et al (eds) Medical robotics and computer assisted surgery. Carnegie Mellon University, Pittsburgh, pp 451–463

Radermacher K, Staudte H-W, Pichler CV, Rau G (1994b) Computerunterstützte Kopplung von Planung und Umsetzung chirurgischer Eingriffe in der Orthopädie. Zeitschrift für Biomedizinische Technik 39:205–206

Radermacher K, Staudte H-W, Rau G (1995) technique for better execution of CT-scan planned orthopedic surgery on bone structures. In: Lemke HU et al (eds) Computer assisted radiology. Springer, Berlin Heidelberg New York, pp 933–938

Radermacher K, Bliem R, Hennecke C, Staudte H-W, Rau G (1996a) DISOS – -A desktop image-processing system for computer assisted orthopedic surgery. In: Weghorst SJ,

Sieburg HB, Morgan K (eds) MMVR 4: Health care in the information age – future tools for transforming Medicine. IOS Press, Amsterdam, pp 675–680

Radermacher K, Rau G, Staudte H-W (1996b) Computer integrated orthopedic surgery – connection of planning and execution in surgical intervention. In: Taylor R, Lavallée S, Burdea GC, Moesges R (eds) Computer integrated surgery. MIT Press, Cambridge (MA), pp 451–463

Radermacher K, Portheine F, Zimolong A, Eichhorn C, Staudte H-W, Rau G (1997a) Image guided orthopedic surgery using individual templates. Experimental results and aspects of the development of a demonstrator for pelvis surgery. In: Troccaz J, Grimson E, Mösges R (eds) CVRMED II and MRCAS III. Lecture Notes in Computer Science, vol. 1205. Springer, Berlin Heidelberg New York, pp 606–616

Radermacher K, Rau G, Staudte H-W (1997b) Computerintegrierte operative Eingriffe in der Orthopädie: Möglichkeiten auch in der Endoprothetik? In: Wessinghage D (ed) Praktische Orthopädie, Bd. 27, Thieme Verlag, Stuttgart, pp 149–164

Radermacher K, Portheine F, Anton M, Zimolong A, Kaspers G, Rau G, Staudte H-W (1998) Computer assisted orthopaedic surgery with image-based individual templates. J Clin Orthop Relat Res 354:28–38

Radermacher K, Portheine F, Schkommodau E, Staudte H-W, Rau G (1999) Entwicklung eines integrierten Planungs- und Fertigungssystems für CT-Bild-basierte individuelle Bearbeitungsschablonen in der orthopädischen Chirurgie. VDI Fortschritts-Berichte 17:56–57

Radermacher K, Kaspers G, Portheine F, Schkommodau E, Staudte H-W (2000a) Klinische Erfahrungen mit der computerunterstützten Planung und intraoperativen Führung mit individuellen Bearbeitungsschablonen für die periacetabuläre Umstellungsosteotomie. Zeitschrift für Biomedizinische Technik 45:204–205

Radermacher K, Portheine F, Schkommodau E (2000b) Rechnerbasierte Entscheidungs-unterstützung zur Planung von Kontaktflächen zur manuellen Referenzierung mit Individualschablonen. Zeitschrift für Biomedizinische Technik 45:227–228

Radermacher K, Wu T, Zimolong A, Cinquin P, Grange S, Niethard FU, Rau G (2001) Netzbasierte Module für Ausbildung, Training und Dokumentation in der Orthopädischen Chirurgie: VOEU. Zeitschrift für Biomedizinische Technik 46:364–365

Rau G, Radermacher K (1997) Operationsplanung und -ausführung in der computerunterstützten Chirurgie. Zeitschrift für Biomedizinische Technik [Suppl 2]:305–306

Rau G, von Pichler C, Radermacher K (1995) Surgical reality. Medical Technology International, Cornhill Publications, London, pp 46–51

Schiffers N, Schkommodau E, Portheine F, Radermacher K, Staudte H-W (2000) Planung und Ausführung von orthopädischen Operationen mit Hilfe von Individualschablonen. Der Orthopäde 29:636–640

Schkommodau E, Klapper U, Birnbaum K, Radermacher K, Staudte H-W (2000) Computerunterstützte Implantation von Pedikelschrauben mit Hilfe von Individualschablonen in der Orthopädischen Chirurgie. Zeitschrift für Biomedizinische Technik 45:206–207

Schkommodau E, Kaspers G, Klapper U, Radermacher K, Staudte H-W (2001) Klinische Erfahrung mit der Individualschablonentechnik. Orthopädische Praxis 37:19–22

Schkommodau E, Decker N, Klapper U, Birnbaum K, Staudte H-W, Radermacher K (2002) Pedikelschraubenimplantation mit dem DISOS-Schablonensystem. In: Konermann W, Haaker R (eds) Navigation und Robotic in der gelenk- und Wirbelsäulenchirurgie. Springer, Berlin Heidelberg New York, pp 395–399

Schkommodau E, Decker N, Klapper U, Birnbaum K, Staudte H-W, Radermacher K (2003) Pedicle screw implantation using the DISOS template system. In: Stiehl JB, Konermann WH, Haaker RG (eds) Navigation and robotics in total joint and spine surgery. Springer, Berlin Heidelberg New York, pp. 501–505

Staudte H-W, Radermacher K, Rau G (1997) CT-abgeleitete Operationsschablone am Beispiel der Tripel-Osteotomie nach Tönnis. In: Wessinghage D (ed) Praktische Orthopädie, Bd. 27, Thieme Verlag, Stuttgart, pp 165–171

Staudte H-W, Radermacher K, Rau G (1998) Computerunterstützte Operationsplanung und -ausführung mit individuellen Bearbeitungsschablonen. Zeitschrift für Orthopädie 136:124–125

Staudte H-W, Schkommodau E, Honscha M, Portheine F, Radermacher R (2002) Beckenosteotomie mit Schablonennavigation. In: Konermann W, Haaker R (2002) Navigation und Robotik in der Gelenk- und Wirbelsäulenchirurgie. Springer, Berlin Heidelberg New York, pp 356–364

Staudte H-W, Schkommodau E, Portheine F, Radermacher K (2003) Pelvic osteotomy with template navigation. In: Stiehl JB, Konermann WH, Haaker RG (eds) Navigation and robotics in total joint and spine surgery. Springer, Berlin Heidelberg New York, pp 455–463

Taylor RH, Mittelstadt BD, Paul HA, Hamson W, Kazanides P, Zahars JH, Williamson B, Musits BL, Glassman E, Bargar WL (1996) An image-directed robotic system for precise orthopaedic surgery. In: Taylor RH, Lavallée St, Burdea GC et al (eds) Computer integrated surgery. MIT Press, Cambridge (MA), pp 379–396

Individual Templates in Total Knee Arthroplasty

Patient-Specific Instruments for Total Knee Replacement: Based on MRI and Whole-Leg Radiograms (VISIONAIRE™)

Carsten O. Tibesku

The VISIONAIRE^{TM} (Smith & Nephew) patient-specific instrumentation is based on a magnetic resonance imaging (MRI) scan of the knee and a whole-leg standing radiogram for calculation of the axes. The preoperative planning is based on the surgeon's individual preferences and can still be changed during the planning process. The surgeon can more easily control the whole-leg standing radiogram measurements than the axes that are calculated from computed tomography (CT) or MRI data. VISIONAIRE^{TM} instruments already include the cutting slots and are fully compatible with conventional instruments, in case the surgeon wishes to change any parameters during surgery.
Experience with this technique has shown a precise fit of the instruments on the articular surfaces and a reliable preoperative sizing of the implants. The scientific literature available is still sparse but shows strong evidence of reduced variability in the long-leg axis as well as improved rotational alignment of the implants. Despite the extra costs incurred for the diagnostics and the disposable instruments, cost-effectiveness is achieved if the time saved is used to perform additional procedures.

Patient-specific instrumentation was introduced in total knee arthroplasty (TKA) to improve implant positioning and decrease the surgery and set-up time in the operating room. Although still the standard of care, conventional manual instruments have failed to achieve consistent implant positioning (Iorio et al. 2012). Navigation has been used for several years to improve implant positioning. So far, it has been shown that there are no differences between conventional instruments and navigated surgery with regards to the mean long-leg axis, but the number of outliers of more than 3° or 5° from a straight leg axis has been shown to be significantly reduced by navigation (Bauwens et al. 2007; Dattani et al. 2009). Imageless navigation was not able to improve rotational alignment for the tibial or femoral components (Cheng et al. 2011; Matziolis et al. 2007), as the manual identification of rotational alignment landmarks during surgery can lead to errors of up to 23° (Jerosch et al. 2002).

The VISIONAIRE^{TM} patient-specific instrumentation is based on medical imaging and has been developed to improve frontal plane and rotational alignment of TKA, as well as to improve the time and cost-efficiency of TKA surgeries.

3.1 Description of VISIONAIRE^{TM} Technology

VISIONAIRE^{TM} patient-specific instruments are based on the data of an MRI of the knee joint and a whole-leg standing radiogram. The frontal plane alignment is based on the mechanical axis, measured off the long-leg standing x-ray, since this is still regarded the gold standard for a successful clinical outcome and long-term survivorship (Lombardi et al. 2011). The MRI consists in a sagittal two-dimensional (2D) sequence requiring about 10 min.

The surgeon needs to provide the preferred anatomical landmarks and principles for the component placement. These principles are essentially the same as for conventional surgery, e.g., up- or downsizing in case of size mismatch, preferred rotational landmark, varus–valgus alignment, thickness of bone resection, and preferred tibial slope.

The images, MRI and whole-leg standing radiogram, are uploaded via the Internet and then monitored for resolution quality and patient motion. The MRI is then segmented to capture all femur/tibia bone and cartilage. The segmented bone and cartilage slices are put together in a 3D model to get the most accurate remodeling of the patient's knee anatomy. An engineer plans a virtual intramedullary rod into the 3D model. Afterwards, the engineer overlies and matches the 3D model with the x-ray image, ensuring proper mechanical alignment. 3D cutting blocks are then imported and matched to the patients' knee anatomy to ensure a proper fit.

An initial proposal on implant positioning according to the above-mentioned preferences is made by the engineer and uploaded to a website. The surgeon receives e-mail notification to check the preoperative planning. At this stage, the surgeon can still decide to change any parameter. After the surgeon's approval, the blocks are manufactured and shipped sterile to the hospital. The femoral patient-specific cutting block includes all the 3D information for component positioning: varus-valgus alignment, anteroposterior positioning, size, flexion,

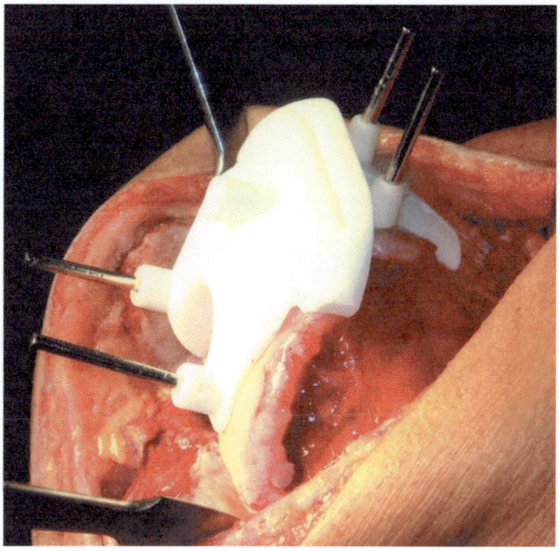

■ **Fig. 3.1** The femoral patient-specific cutting block is fixed to the articular surface. Note the fit of the block on the articular surface

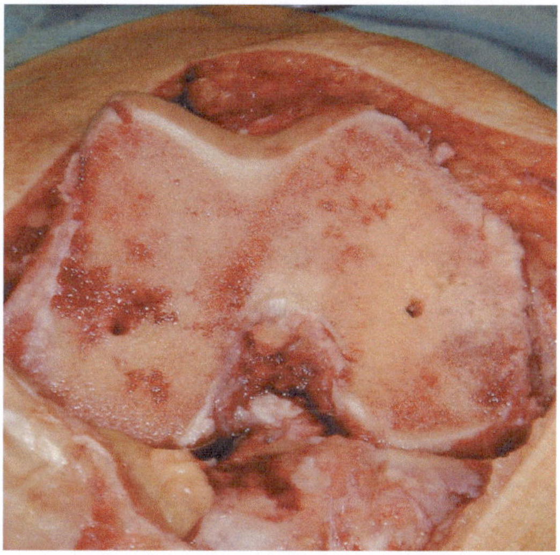

■ **Fig. 3.2** The distal femoral cut is made. Note the drill/pin holes on the bone surface that will receive the 4-in-1 cutting block

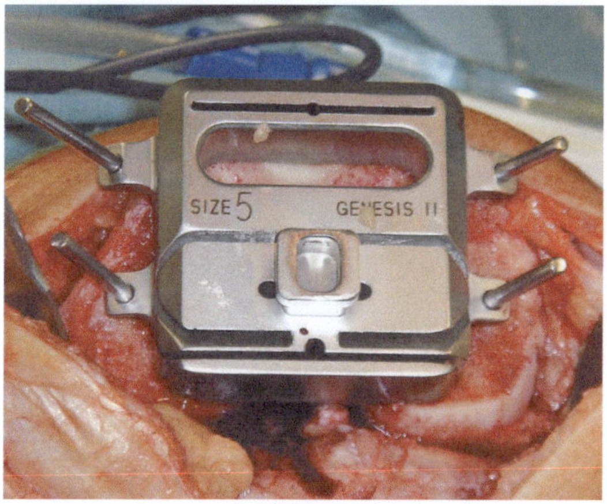

■ **Fig. 3.3** The 4-in-1 cutting block is applied to the predrilled pin holes on the distal femoral bone cut. The VISIONAIRE™ patient-specific femoral cutting block contains all the information on the size, flexion, anteroposterior positioning, and rotation of the femoral component

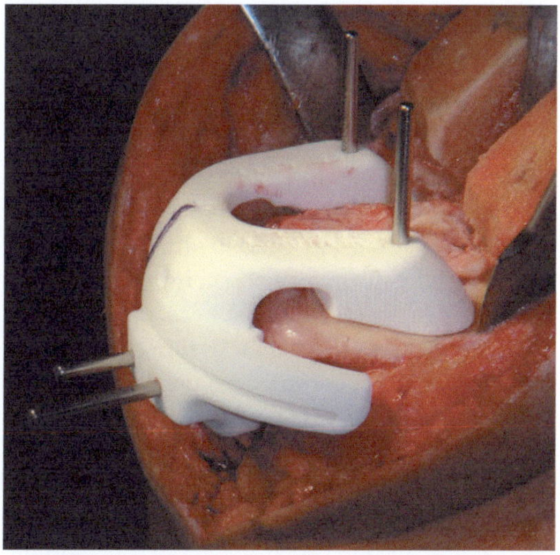

■ **Fig. 3.4** The tibial patient-specific cutting block is fixed to the articular surface

rotation, and all resection thicknesses. The same applies to the tibial patient-specific cutting block: varus-valgus alignment, anteroposterior and mediolateral positioning, size, slope, and rotation.

As the database for the cutting blocks consists of MRI data, it offers a unique fit of blocks to the bone (■ Fig. 3.1, Fig. 3.2, Fig. 3.3, Fig. 3.4). Bony structures as well as the remaining cartilage and the osteophytes are built into the design of the blocks to ensure a custom fit.

The blocks are made from medical-grade nylon by laser sintering. In contrast to milling, this ensures a smooth surface for a perfect fit. All instruments include size, patient name, patient side, and TKA system name, as well as reference markings to ensure proper fit and alignment (epicondylar axis and anteroposterior axis at the femur and medial 1/3 tibial tubercle at the tibia). The pin holes used to fix the patient-specific instruments to the bone are compatible with standard instrumentation, in case the surgeon needs to change intraoperatively. The blocks are sterile packed and can be sterilized up to three times if necessary.

Currently, VISIONAIRE™ blocks are available for the Journey BCS, TC Plus, Legion Primary, and Genesis II total knee systems, for both cruciate retaining and posterior stabilized implants.

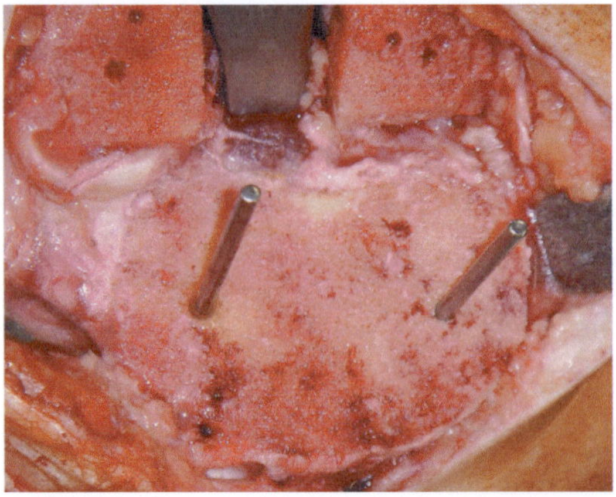

Fig. 3.5 The tibial bone cut is made. Note the drill/pin holes on the bone surface that will receive size-specific instruments

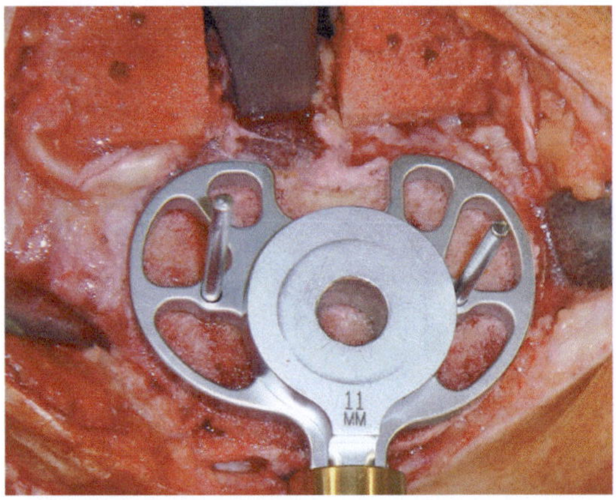

Fig. 3.6 The size-specific tibial instrument for stem preparation is slipped onto the predrilled pins. The VISIONAIRE™ patient-specific tibial cutting block contains all the information on the size, slope, anteroposterior and mediolateral positioning, and rotation of the tibial component

3.2 Intraoperative Use

In contrast to any other patient-specific instrumentation, the VISIONAIRE™ blocks are not only a pin positioning guide for conventional cutting blocks, but also include the cutting slots. This means that the oscillating saw is guided by the nylon slot, and there is no need for a change of instruments after setting the pins.

First, the patient-specific femoral cutting block is applied to the articular surface. The pin holes are then drilled, beginning with the distal hole, and the pins are placed with a hammer (Fig. 3.1). Both distal drill holes will receive the 4-in-1 cutting block after the distal cut has been made. Both anterior pins are compatible with the conventional distal cutting block, in case there is need for additional distal resection, e.g., if there is flexion contracture.

After the distal cut has been performed (Fig. 3.2), the pins of the 4-in-1 cutting block are placed into the predrilled holes on the distal bone cut (Fig. 3.3). This means that the patient-specific femoral cutting blocks contain all the information on the size, flexion, anteroposterior positioning, and rotation of the femoral component.

The tibial block is then applied onto the articular surface and the anteromedial tibia and the pin holes are predrilled and the pins placed with a hammer (Fig. 3.4). Both anteromedial pins are compatible with the conventional tibial cutting block, in case additional proximal tibial resection is needed. After the tibial cut has been made, the pins are placed into the predrilled holes on the bone surface (Fig. 3.5). The size-specific tibial instrument for stem preparation is slipped onto the predrilled pins (Fig. 3.6). This means that the patient-specific tibial cutting block contains all the information on the size, slope, anteroposterior and mediolateral positioning, and rotation of the tibial component.

Both femoral and tibial cutting blocks include lines to conventionally evaluate rotation, and a long drop rod that fits into the cutting slots is available to check the alignment before any cuts are made.

After the bone cuts have been made, a trial reduction is carried out and the necessary steps of ligament balancing are performed.

3.3 Limitations

All contraindications to the use of MRI are limitations of patient-specific instrumentation: metal implants around the knee, pacemaker, claustrophobia, severe obesity. Additionally, the quality of the whole-leg standing radiogram with regard to true anteroposterior projection and avoidance of malrotation needs to be addressed. If a true anteroposterior whole-leg standing radiogram cannot be obtained, e.g., in severe flexion contracture, separate anteroposterior radiograms of the tibia and the femur can be used.

3.4 Early Experience and First Published Results

The author started using the VISIONAIRE^{TM} patient-specific instrumentation in October 2009, and has performed more than 150 procedures to date. In all cases, the Genesis II PS TKA system was used.

An analysis of intraoperative findings was made for the first 131 cases (82 males, 49 females). The patients' mean age was 67 years (range, 26–88 years). In 97 cases there was varus osteoarthritis (OA), in 7 cases patellofemoral OA, in 15 cases valgus OA, and 11 cases were of posttraumatic or postinfection nature. Three of these cases had a history of high tibial osteotomy. In 12 cases a patella replacement was performed, in 119 cases the patella was left unreplaced. Twenty-eight cases required a lateral patellar release (3× grade 1, 19× grade 4, 5× grade 5, 1× grade 6). A medial release was required in 37 of the knees (13× grade 1, 6× grade 2a, 11× grade 2b, 6× grade 3, 1× grade 4) and a release of the lateral structures was required in 17 knees (12× grade 1, 5×grade 2). The length of surgery was 52 min on average (range, 35–86 min).

It was always possible to find a good fit of the femoral block; in four cases the tibial block was abandoned because of a lack of fit to the articular surface. All of these cases occurred during the first 30 surgeries and should be attributed to the author's learning curve. In all of the cases, the femoral sizing was accurate. In 24 cases (18%), the size of the tibial component was changed during operation (6 smaller, 18 larger than planned). There was no need to change the rotation (neither tibial nor femoral) or the tibial slope. The radiological and clinical outcome of these patients is currently being evaluated.

3.5 Clinical Results

So far, there are only sparse reports in the literature on the clinical or radiological outcome of TKA using patient-specific instrumentation. Nunley and colleagues reported that conventional instrumentation and patient-specific instrumentation based on whole-leg MRI data and aiming for the mechanical axis (Signature, Biomet) achieved similar percentages of outliers from a straight leg axis (40% and 32%) (Nunley et al. 2012b). Furthermore, patient-specific instrumentation based on whole-leg MRI data and aiming for the kinematic axis (Otismed) resulted in 64% of valgus outliers from a straight leg axis (Nunley et al. 2012b). Using the same system, Ng and coworkers found fewer outliers from the neutral leg axis (Ng et al. 2012).

Only one study used the VISIONAIRE^{TM} patient-specific instrumentation that is based on a whole-leg standing radiogram (Noble et al. 2012). Noble and coworkers compared 15 VISIONAIRE^{TM} patient-specific instrumentation TKAs with 14 conventional TKAs using the Legion knee system. They reported a postoperative mechanical alignment significantly closer to zero in the VISIONAIRE^{TM} group than in the conventional group (1.7° vs. 2.8°), as well as significantly reduced operating time and number of instrument trays used (Noble et al. 2012).

In a radiological evaluation of the first 100 total knee replacements done with VISIONAIRE^{TM}, the author evaluated the frontal plane alignment of the whole leg (Daniilidis and Tibesku 2013). The average hip-knee-angle (HKA) changed from 175.5±5.6° preoperatively to 178.5±1.7° postoperatively. The rate of ±3° and ±5° HKA outliers was 11% and 3%, respectively. The mechanical axis passed through the central third of the knee in the majority of cases (93 knees, 93%). In conclusion, the use of VISIONAIRE^{TM} technology was able to achieve a neutral mechanical axis on average in patients undergoing TKA.

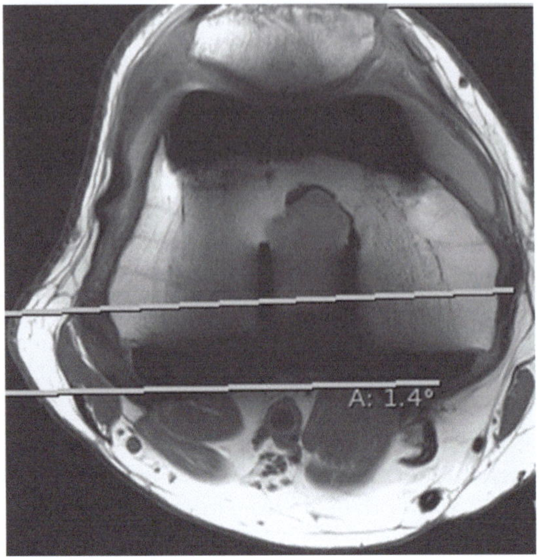

Fig. 3.7 Axial MRI scan of the oxinium femoral component of a Genesis II TKA with measurement of the angle between the transepicondylar axis and posterior condylar line. The use of patient-specific instruments reduced the number of outliers from perfect rotational alignment from 20% to 2%

3.6 Rotational Alignment

Besides the long axes, the VISIONAIRE™ system aims at reducing outliers in the so-called short axes, as in rotational alignment of the femoral and tibial components. In a cadaver experiment, VISIONAIRE™ patient-specific instrumentation achieved a mean femoral external rotation of 1.6° (SD 2.6°; Tibesku et al. 2012b). It was also shown that CT-based patient-specific instrumentation can lead to outliers in rotational alignment (Tibesku et al. 2012b).

In a recent study, the rotational alignment of femoral components was evaluated (Heyse and Tibesku 2012). An MRI analysis of 94 patients following TKA was conducted (Fig. 3.7). All surgeries were performed by the author. Of these, 46 operations were carried out using VISIONAIRE™ patient-specific instrumentation and 48 using conventional instrumentation. The rotation of the femoral components was determined in the MRI group and deviations of more than 3° were considered outliers. There were significantly more outliers in the conventional (22.9%) group than in the patient-specific instrumentation group (2.2%, p=0.003). In this set-up, VISIONAIRE™ patient-specific instrumentation was effective in significantly reducing outliers of optimal rotational femoral component alignment during TKA (Heyse and Tibesku 2012).

3.7 Cost-Effectiveness

Besides the improvements in accuracy, patient-specific instruments lead to different procedures in the operating room and sterilization department. The VISIONAIRE™ patient-specific instruments eliminate as many as 22 steps associated with conventional instrumentation. The number of trays that need to be sterilized and set up before operation can be reduced from six to two/three for a Genesis PS knee system. This leads to an inventory reduction for hospitals and companies.

In the near future, all instruments will become available as disposable (Fig. 3.8). Using these instruments, the number of trays of conventional instruments will be reduced to only one. These measures in turn will reduce the time needed for surgery and OR set-up as well as the time and costs for sterilization and clean up. On the other hand, the cost of the procedure is increased by the additional MRI and the patient-specific instruments. So far, reports in the literature have been inconsistent as to whether the use of patient-specific instrumentation can reduce the overall costs for a TKA (Slover and Tibesku 2012; Nunley et al. 2012a; Watters et al. 2011). In our own study, we evaluated the benefits of using patient-specific instrumentation in an activity-based costing (ABC) model (Tibesku et al. 2012a). This analysis suggests that VISIONAIRE™ patient-specific instrumentation is an economically effective method in TKA. The use of patient-specific instrumentation can lead to incremental revenue for the hospital, on the condition that time savings are effectively used to perform more procedures. The additional revenue will offset the higher costs associated with cutting blocks and diagnostics (Tibesku et al. 2012a).

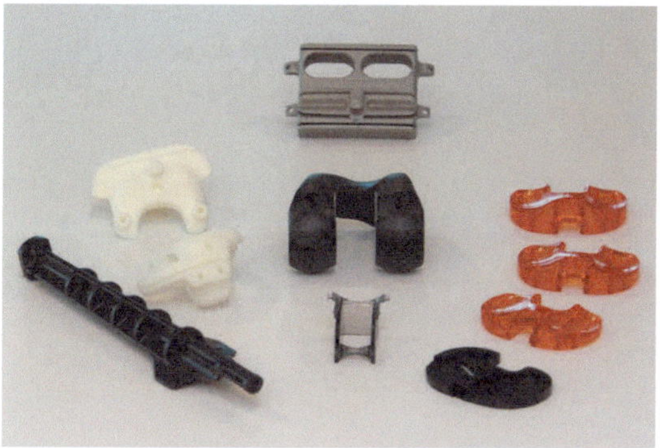

Fig. 3.8 In the near future, the sterile box will include not only the patient-specific instruments, but also size-specific disposable 4-in-1 femoral blocks and trials. This means that all preparation steps can be carried out with this set and there is no need for conventional instruments

3.8 Future Outlook

In the near future, all instruments will become available as disposable and will reduce the number of trays of conventional instruments to only one. The next step of individualization is the combination of more than one standard implant in the same knee using patient-specific instrumentation, e.g., combined medial unicompartmental and patellofemoral arthroplasty. The final step will be the use of patient-specific instrumentation with patient-specific implants. Since the important parameters of individualization of a knee replacement (anatomical or kinematic) are not yet known, this development will need more basic research in the future.

References

Bauwens K, Matthes G, Wich M, Gebhard F, Hanson B, Ekkernkamp A, Stengel D (2007) Navigated total knee replacement. A meta-analysis. J Bone Joint Surg Am 89:261-269

Cheng T, Zhang G, Zhang X (2011) Imageless navigation system does not improve component rotational alignment in total knee arthroplasty. J Surg Res 171:590–600

Daniilidis K, Tibesku CO (2013) Frontal plane alignment after total knee arthroplasty using patient-specific instruments. Int Orthop 37:45–50

Dattani R, Patnaik S, Kantak A, Tselentakis G (2009) Navigation knee replacement. Int Orthop 33:7–10

Heyse TJ, Tibesku CO (2012) Improved femoral component rotation in TKA using patient-specific instrumentation. Knee [Epub ahead of print]

Iorio R, Bolle G, Conteduca F, Valeo L, Conteduca J, Mazza D, Ferretti A (2012) Accuracy of manual instrumentation of tibial cutting guide in total knee arthroplasty. Knee Surg Sports Traumatol Arthrosc [Epub ahead of print]

Jerosch J, Peuker E, Philipps B, Filler T (2002) Interindividual reproducibility in perioperative rotational alignment of femoral components in knee prosthetic surgery using the transepicondylar axis. Knee Surg Sports Traumatol Arthrosc 10:194–197

Lombardi AV Jr, Berend KR, Ng VY (2011) Neutral mechanical alignment: a requirement for successful TKA: affirms. Orthopedics 34:e504–506

Matziolis G, Krocker D, Weiss U, Tohtz S, Perka C (2007) A prospective, randomized study of computer-assisted and conventional total knee arthroplasty. Three-dimensional evaluation of implant alignment and rotation. J Bone Joint Surg Am 89:236–243

Ng VY, DeClaire JH, Berend KR, Gulick BC, Lombardi AV Jr (2012) Improved accuracy of alignment with patient-specific positioning guides compared with manual instrumentation in TKA. Clin Orthop Rel Res 470:99–107

Noble JW,Jr, Moore CA, Liu N (2012) The value of patient-matched instrumentation in total knee arthroplasty. J Arthrop 27:153–155

Nunley RM, Ellison BS, Ruh EL, Williams BM, Foreman K, Ford AD, Barrack RL (2012a) Are patient-specific cutting blocks cost-effective for total knee arthroplasty? Clin Orthop Rel Res 470:889–894

Nunley RM, Ellison BS, Zhu J, Ruh EL, Howell SM, Barrack RL (2012b) Do patient-specific guides improve coronal alignment in total knee arthroplasty? Clin Orthop Rel Res 470:895–902

Slover JD, Rubash HE, Malchau H, Bosco JA (2012) Cost-effectiveness analysis of custom total knee cutting blocks. J Arthrop 27:180–185

Tibesku CO, Hofer P, Ruys CJM, Portegies W, Fennema P (2012a) Benefits of using customized intrumentation in total knee arthroplasty: results from an activity based costing model. Arch Orthop Trauma Surg [Epub ahead of print]

Tibesku CO, Innocenti B, Wong P, Salehi A, Labey L (2012b) Can CT-based patient-matched instrumentation achieve consistent rotational alignment in knee arthroplasty? Arch Orthop Trauma Surg 132:171–177

Watters TS, Mather RC 3rd, Browne JA, Berend KR, Lombardi AV Jr, Bolognesi MP (2011) Analysis of procedure-related costs and proposed benefits of using patient-specific approach in total knee arthroplasty. J Surg Orthop Adv 20:112–126

MyKnee®: Patient-Matched Instruments

Stefan Dittrich, Werner Anderl

Proper alignment of the components aimed at accurately reconstructing the mechanical leg axis has gained crucial importance in total knee replacements. Any deviation from the mechanical leg axis by more than 3° varus or valgus will have a negative impact on the outcome (Fang et al. 2009). Computer-assisted surgery (CAS) has markedly improved the accuracy of both component placement and reconstruction of the mechanical leg axis (Fu et al. 2012). Nevertheless, compromises such as extended surgery time and enhanced complication rate, in particular owing to the requirement that additional pins need to be placed, have had to be accepted. These disadvantages of CAS have been eliminated thanks to the development of patient-matched cutting blocks and pin-positioning guides. MyKnee® by Medacta was one of the first systems of this type available on the international market (Koch2010).

4.1 What Is MyKnee®?

MyKnee® is the extension of a conventional total knee replacement system (GMK®, Global Medacta Knee) that features patient-matched, single-use cutting blocks. These cutting blocks are designed and manufactured using three-dimensional (3D) reconstructions of the patient's knee joint and its corresponding axes, calculated by means of computed tomography (CT) or magnetic resonance imaging (MRI). To create these CT or MRI images, Medacta® provides a special protocol for taking thin-slice scans of the knee and survey scans of the hips and ankles. The planning stage begins after these are uploaded to the website. The uploaded image data are first subjected to a quality control. A technician then begins to plan the surgery, taking into consideration the surgeon's specifications. CT images are particularly suited for exact planning as they allow bony landmarks to be more accurately identified (Victor et al. 2009). After planning is completed, the surgeon can check and selectively modify individual parameters using the 3D planning tool. As soon as the plan is confirmed, the cutting blocks go into production. The blocks are shipped unsterilized and must therefore be sterilized before surgery.

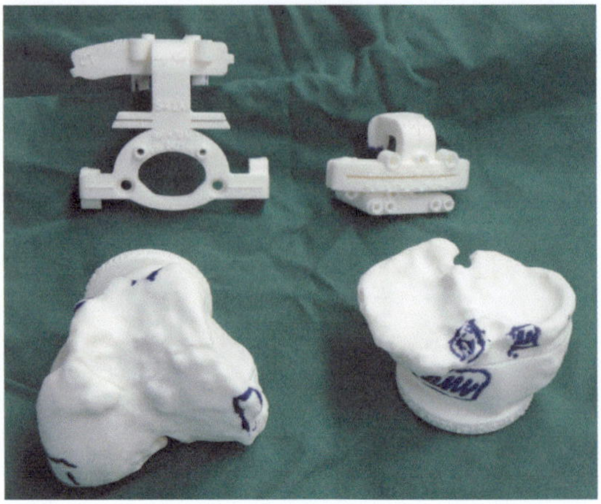

Fig. 4.1 Preoperative check of the cutting blocks and marking of the contact points

4.2 Operative Technique

The surgical access route can be selected variably depending on the surgeon's preference. The cutting blocks are supplied for medial parapatellar, lateral parapatellar, and minimally invasive access. In patients with gonarthrosis without malpositioning or varus gonarthrosis, we prefer the medial parapatellar access, but choose the lateral parapatellar approach when patients present with valgus gonarthrosis. The access route must be specified at the planning stage. Before surgery, the cutting blocks are placed on the individual model (tibia/femur) and the contact points are labeled (Fig. 4.1).

This step facilitates the dissection. Once the access route has been selected, the tibia and femur are exposed. Next, the contact points of the cutting blocks must then be carefully freed of cartilage and other soft tissue (Fig. 4.2). This step is of paramount importance, as the blocks are created using CT images and the calculations are exclusively based on the bony parts. Leaving any cartilage at the contact points could therefore lead to axis deviations of several degrees.

4.2.1 Tibial Cut

We prefer the tibia-first technique; however, it is up to the surgeon to decide whether to use the femur-

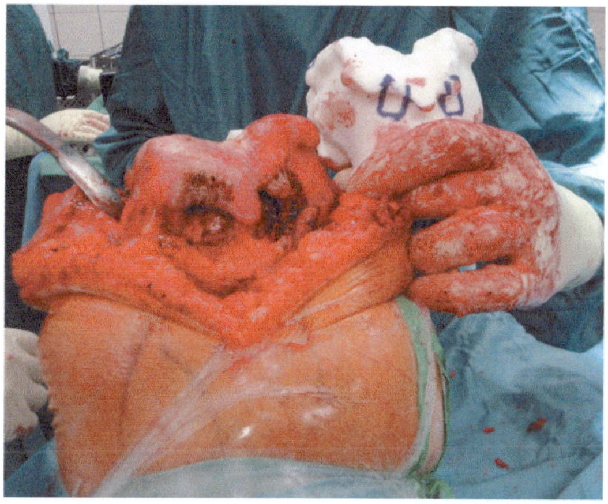

■ **Fig. 4.2** Exact removal of soft tissue at the contact points

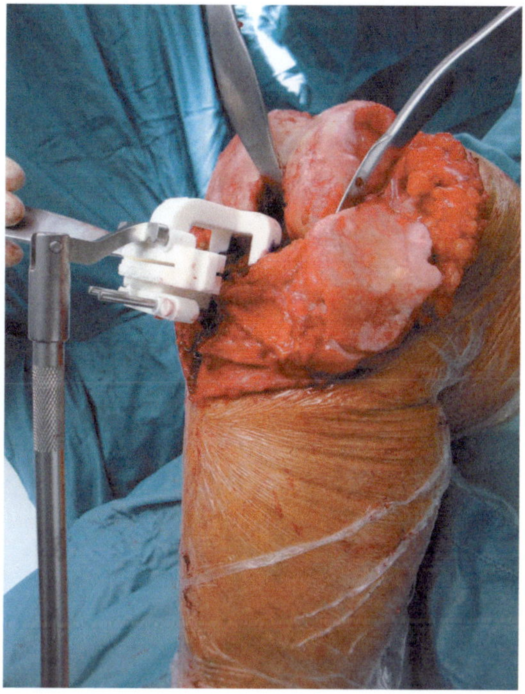

■ **Fig. 4.3** Fixation of the cutting blocks with pins

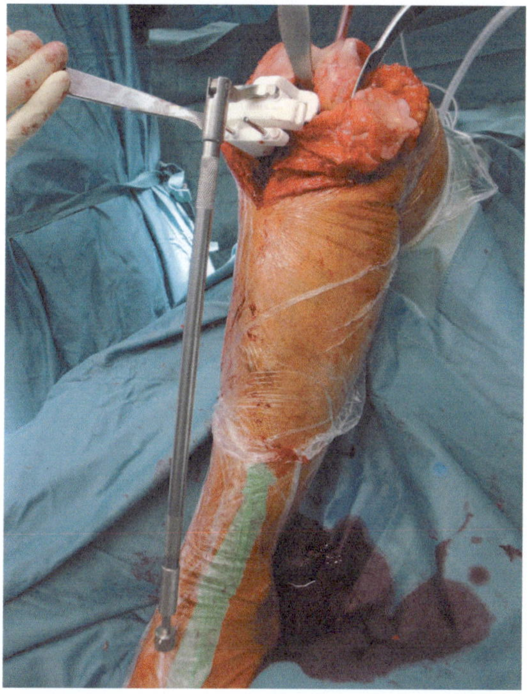

■ **Fig. 4.4** Verification of alignment with alignment guide

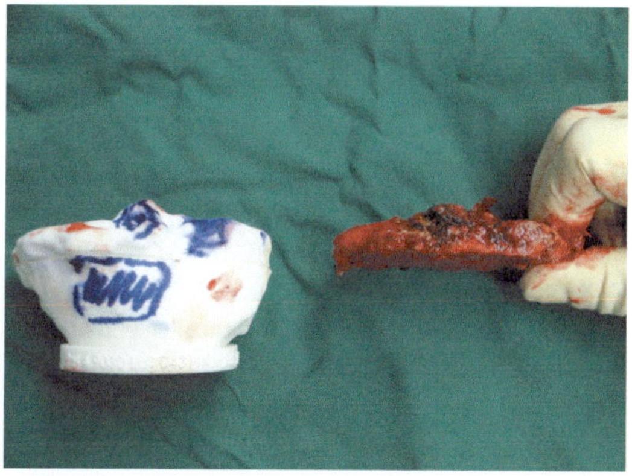

■ **Fig. 4.5** Comparison of resected tissue with resection height on the bone model

first technique. The cutting block is positioned on the patient's tibial plateau; note how important it is that it be perfectly seated on the contact points. Exact positioning results in maximal stability of the block on the tibial plateau. Next, the cutting block is fixed in place with two pins (■ Fig. 4.3) and the alignment checked using a telescopic alignment rod (■ Fig. 4.4). The resection level can also be checked using a sickle finger. Once the positioning is satisfactory, an oblique pin is used to give the block additional stability for the subsequent sawing procedure. The resected tissue can be compared with the resection level on the model (tibia/femur) (■ Fig. 4.5). Now, the oblique pin and the tibial cut-

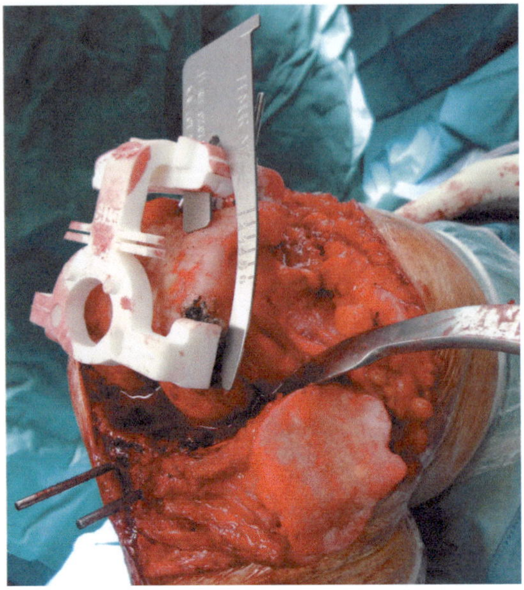

Fig. 4.6 Verification of femoral distal cut with sickle finger

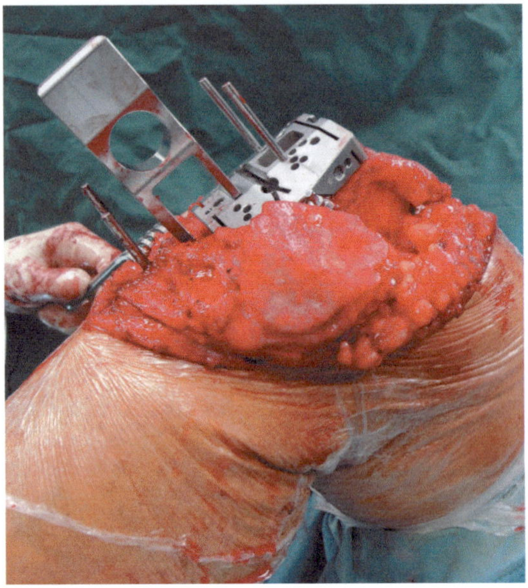

Fig. 4.7 Verification of ligament balance with spacer

ting block are removed. The parallel pins are left in situ to allow for a GMK® standard cutting block to be attached if a postresection is needed.

4.2.2 Femoral Cut

The femoral cutting block is fixed to the femur after repeatedly checking the four contact points – two on the anterior and two on the distal femur. The intended resection can be checked with a sickle finger (Fig. 4.6). Here, too, the stability of the fixed block provides information as to proper positioning. Fixation is performed with three pins. Next, the pin holes on the 4-in-1 block, which also determine the femoral rotation, are pre-drilled distally. The distal cut is then performed and the extension gap checked by means of spacers. As with a tibial cut, a GMK® standard cutting block can be used for a distal femoral cut in case a postresection is needed. The distal pins for the 4-in-1 block are then set and the block (GMK® standard cutting block) is attached. Using a sickle finger, the anterior and posterior cut can now be checked. Ligament balancing in the flexion gap can now be performed with a special flexion gap spacer (Fig. 4.7). The surgeon can then perform a soft-tissue release or postresection according to his or her conventional practice as required for joint stability. Next, femoral and tibial finishing is performed according to the GMK® standard operative technique. The result is checked with the trial implants. After this, the implantation can be accomplished with or without cement.

4.3 The Advantages of MyKnee®

Preoperative planning enables exact positioning of the implants as well as perfect reconstruction of the mechanical leg axis. The CT-based version makes exact surgical planning possible even if metal implants had been used in previous operations. It is thus possible to perfectly plan the switch from a semi-sled to a total knee replacement and minimize bone loss in the process. Even in patients who have undergone medullary nailing of the femur or cruciate ligament reconstruction with metal implants, this poses no obstacle.

Opening the intramedullary canal for intramedullary axis alignment during femoral dissection is no longer necessary and greatly reduces blood loss; packed red blood cells are only required in rare

Tab. 4.1 Advantages of CT vs. MRI

Computed tomography	Magnetic resonance imaging
+ More affordable	+ No radiation
+ Better demarcation of the osteophytes	
+ No contraindications	– More expensive
+ Markedly shorter examination time	– Contraindications
	– Markedly longer examination time
– Radiation exposure	– Artifacts
	– Availability

cases. Two-thirds fewer instruments are required than with the standard armamentarium, which in turn means less instrument preparation time is necessary and sterilization costs are cut dramatically. The implant sizes required for surgery are known beforehand and it is thus possible to significantly reduce inventory.

And, last but not least, the surgery time can also be shortened by reducing the number of operative steps required. We see a clear advantage over pin-positioning guides, as it is not necessary to switch between patient-matched and standard instruments. Also, there is less manipulation in this position. The supplied 3D models of the tibia and femur enable the surgeon to verify both the resection plane and the resection volume. Should the surgeon have doubts about the planning in mid-surgery, a trouble-free switch to conventional instruments and surgical techniques is possible at any time. An added advantage of this surgical technique is the steep learning curve.

Tab. 4.2 CT radiation exposure

	(mSv)
Pelvic survey radiograph	0.7–1
CT of the abdomen and pelvis	15
CT of the pelvis	3–8
CT of the knee	0.16
CT of the ankle	0.07
Thoracic radiograph	0.01
Transatlantic flight	0.1

Average radiation exposure for Austria, 3.0 mSv; for Germany, 2.0 mSv; for Switzerland, 4.0 mSv

4.4 The Disadvantages of MyKnee®

The costs of the cutting blocks and the CT/MRI are offset, to a certain extent, by the savings mentioned above. The preoperative logistics as well as the time necessary to carry out the planning are worth mentioning. They certainly represent additional expenditure in terms of time and money as compared to conventional techniques, which should not be underestimated. The advantages of CT vs. MRI are listed in Tab. 4.1.

Tab. 4.2 lists the radiation exposure of CT imaging.

4.5 Initial Results

In July 2009, the first total knee replacement with the MyKnee® system was implanted in Switzerland (Balgrist Clinic). The first time we used the MyKnee® cutting blocks was in July 2010 in the Department for Orthopedics and Orthopedic Surgery at the hospital »Barmherzige Schwestern« in Vienna. Since then through December 2011, we have implanted 250 total knee replacements by employing the MyKnee® technique. In 243 cases, the mechanical leg axis measurements were within the target range of 180°±3°. In the seven cases outside of this range, the surgeon had intentionally left residual varus/valgus in two cases. As intramedullary drilling is obviated, packed red blood cells were used significantly less often. In one case only were the blocks not used, because examination with the alignment rod showed a significant deviation of the axis despite repeated placement of the tibia cutting block. The surgeon was able to immediately switch to the conventional surgical technique in this case. In three other cases, the conventional technique had to be used after the tibial cut since the femoral cutting block was dropped and only one sterile cutting block was available per patient.

4.6 Conclusion

MyKnee® is a new and innovative surgical technique with a steep learning curve. The results obtained are at least consistent with the level of computer-navigated versions; at the same time, surgery times are significantly reduced and fewer surgical instruments are needed. At a minimum, MyKnee® mechanical leg axis reconstruction and component placement are equally as exact. We consider MyKnee® to be a reliable system for the implantation of total knee replacements, featuring the advantage of precise preoperative computer-assisted 3D planning by CT/MRI.

References

Fang DM, Ritter MA, Davis KE (2009) Coronal alignment in total knee arthroplasty. Just how important is it? J Arthroplasty 24 [Suppl 1]:39–43

Fu Y, Wang M, Liu Y, Fu Q (2012) Alignment outcomes in navigated total knee arthroplasty: a meta-analysis. Knee Surg Sports Traumatol Arthrosc 20:1075–1082

Koch PP (2010) Patient matched instrumentation MyKnee® system: a new vision in total knee replacement. Maitrise Orthopedique 198

Victor J, Van Doninck D, Labey L, Innocenti B, Parizel PM, Bellemans J (2009) How precise can bony landmarks be determined on a CT scan of the knee? Knee 16:358–365

Zimmer® Patient-Specific Instruments for Total and Unicompartmental Knee Replacement

Georg Köster

The current outcome of total knee replacement is acceptable, but many attempts have been made to improve the results. The demand for improvement is high, as many goals need to be realized. Good clinical function and longevity are based on correct positioning of the components in coronal, sagittal, and axial planes as well as on soft tissue balancing in flexion and extension, joint line reconstruction, and correct patella tracking. Computer-assisted navigation has resulted in improved alignment but has neither eliminated outliers nor improved the clinical outcome. Navigation during surgery is time consuming and the intraoperative reproducibility of the landmarks varies. Nevertheless, it is widely accepted that coronal, sagittal, and axial alignment is an important factor in the overall result in total knee replacement. Malalignment could be related to instability, persistent pain, and stiffness as well as – in the long term – to wear, osteolysis, and loosening. The goal of patient-specific instrumentation (PSI) technology is to plan and control the several degrees of alignment before or during surgery in order to increase accuracy and improve handling as well as logistics.

5.1 Principle

Based on preoperative magnetic resonance imaging (MRI) of the hip, knee, and ankle, a three-dimensional (3D) model of the patient's anatomy is created. The anatomical 3D model is used to simulate and evaluate implant placement and to generate a default preoperative plan. The planning software enables the surgeon to modify this plan and to vary the implant family, implant brand, component size, and positioning in axial, sagittal, and coronal views. A cartilage mapping allows the surgeon to review the cartilage thickness. This may support the decision between implantation of a unicompartmental knee replacement (UNI) and total knee replacement (TKA) in certain cases. After approval of the surgical planning, disposable patient-matched pin placement guides (TKA) or cutting blocks (UNI) are manufactured for the femur and tibia to be used during surgery. The pins that are placed intraoperatively with the customized guiding instruments can be used for placement of the conventional instrumentation. This allows for adaptations according to the intraoperative findings and flexibility concerning the surgical technique.

5.2 Indications

The use of Zimmer® PSI is indicated for patients in whom an implantation of a TKA or UNI is planned. Currently, the system can be used with certain implants only. In TKA these implants include Zimmer® NexGen CR and NexGen CR-Flex fixed bearing, Zimmer® NexGen LPS and LPS-Flex fixed bearing and the corresponding Gender Solution implants, as well as Zimmer® Gender Solutions NaturalKnee Flex fixed bearing prostheses. In UNI, Zimmer® Unicompartmental High Flex Knee System prostheses are included.

5.3 Contraindications/Constraints

Patients must be excluded from the use of Zimmer® PSI if they suffer from an infection of the knee joint, if metal objects are located within a distance of 150 mm from the joint line, and if patients are unable to undergo an MRI scan or if it is not possible to perform MRI according to the scan protocol with an acceptable quality. Reasons that might impede making an MRI scan with acceptable quality are:

1. The patient is in pain or has a pathology that makes it impossible to keep the leg still during the entire examination, causing motion artifacts in the images.
2. The patient is not allowed to undergo an MRI examination (e.g., the patient has a pacemaker, aneurysm clips in the brain, metal objects in the body that are not compatible with MRI).
3. The patient is too obese, which makes the use of the appropriate coils during the MRI examination impossible.
4. The patient has certain intra- or extra-articular deformations.

Intra-articular deformations can have two different impacts on the PSI system. Firstly, the correct position of the anatomical landmarks can be compromised, which can have an effect on the reference coordinate system and therefore on the correct placement of the implants. The impact of this should be evaluated on a patient-by-patient basis. For example, a deformation of the anterior trochlea can make the femoral anteroposterior (AP) axis unreliable as a rotation reference, but it does not impact other rotation references. Severely degenerated tibia plateaus can compromise placement of the tibial guide.

Secondly, intra-articular deformations, such as large osteophytes within the contact area of the PSI guide on the bone, can compromise the contact surface between the bone/cartilage and the Zimmer® PSI guide so that it is impossible to produce a set of PSI guides according to the standard PSI design that guarantees a sufficient and stable bone/cartilage contact. Also, the applicability of Zimmer® PSI should be judged on a patient-by-patient basis. Extra-articular deformations have an impact on the overall alignment of the entire leg. In general, extra-articular deformations cause the knee joint to be misaligned with respect to the mechanical axis. Because of this, the orientation of the reference coordinate system linked to the femur or tibia becomes unreliable and the implant position and orientation are compromised.

5.4 Preoperative Process

To prepare a case for PSI, a specific process flow has to be followed. Once a patient has been selected, the surgeon creates the case using a special online management system (OMS). A scan date for the MRI is scheduled at a previously qualified medical imaging center. After scanning, the images are sent to Materialise, a company that supplies the software and is responsible for processing the images, creating the 3D models, and producing the guides. A quality check of the images is followed by segmentation and creation of a 3D model. Using this bone model, simulation and evaluation of implant placement are performed and a default preoperative plan is generated. The plan is forwarded to the surgeon, who has to check, adjust, and finally approve the plan before sending it back. Materialise designs a 3D pin placement (TKA) or cutting guide (UNI) and, if required, a 3D bone model of the tibia and femur using CAD software. Subsequently, they manufacture the parts and ship them to Zimmer, which then forwards them to the hospital.

The current status of the workflow can be tracked online at any time.

5.5 Planning

The planner allows the surgeon to simulate the placement of the implants and the corresponding resections in TKA and UNI knee replacement surgery. It provides an adapted graphical user interface that displays the data needed to complete the preoperative planning by means of 2D views where surgical parameters can be adjusted and where measurements can be verified. A 3D view displays the 3D anatomical bone models, the landmarks that were used to define the default plan, the cut bone surfaces, and the implant overlay on the bone surfaces.

The femur and tibia planning sections provide 2D information on the position of the cut planes and anatomical references, including the mechanical axis. The 3D view displays information on anatomical landmarks, on cut surfaces according to the 2D parameters, and on the final result with the implant in place. The femur and tibia can be viewed independently. All bones are shown with cartilage.

5.5.1 Planning Total Knee Replacement

In total knee replacement, after inspection of the proposed planning, the selection and determination of the preferred femur and tibia implant are performed by viewing the 3D cut surfaces and implant overlays. It is recommended to start with the femur implant brand and size, since the availability of the tibia implants depends on the selected femur implant (◘ Fig. 5.1a–e).

The femoral planning consists of three 2D views, each aligned with one of the anatomical planes and the femoral mechanical axis. In the coronal view, which is vertically aligned, the distal resection depth and varus/valgus angle can be adjusted. The axial view of the femur is aligned horizontally with the epicondylar line. Posterior resection and

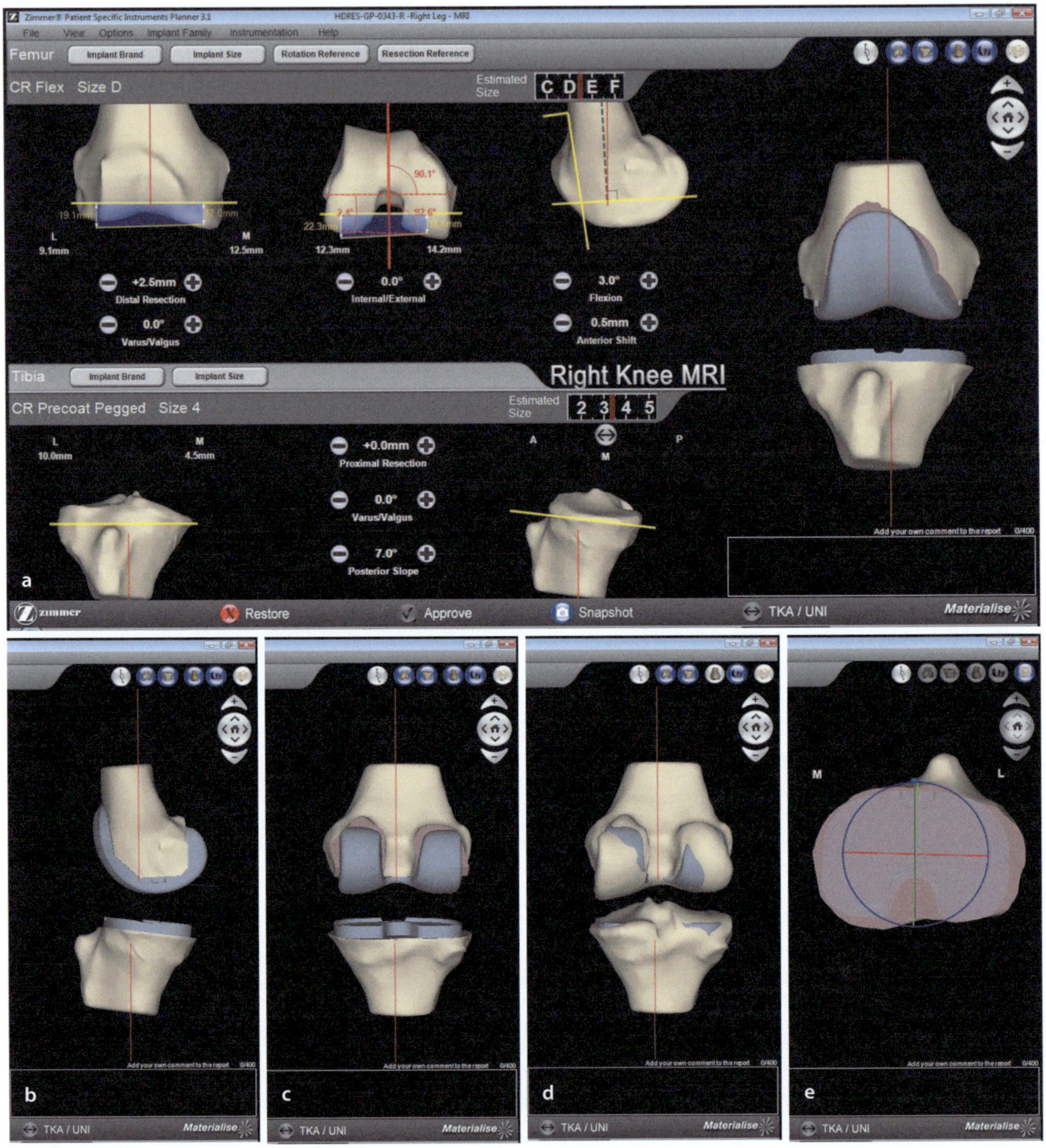

■ **Fig. 5.1a–e** Display for planning total knee replacement. The default preoperative plan can be modified with respect to the different parameters in the coronal, axial, and sagittal view (**a**). The 3D model on the *right* can be rotated horizontally and vertically. It shows the implant with cut surfaces from the different perspectives (**a, b, c**) or the implant covered by the bone (**d**). Several views can be selected: implant with cut surfaces, the cut surfaces only, the implant covered by the bone without cut surfaces, or the bone model only with the landmarks. The posterior view provides an additional orientation to help find the correct resection depth that influences the flexion gap. Looking on the tibia from above (**e**) helps determine the proper size, coverage, and orientation of the component

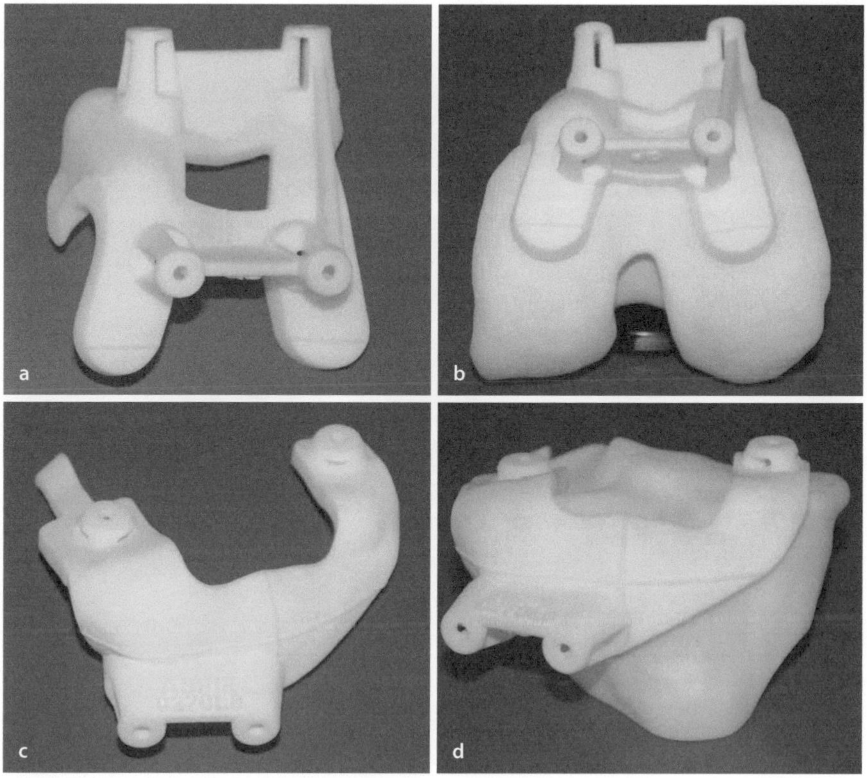

Fig. 5.2a–d Femoral and tibial pin guide for total knee replacement (**a, c**) can be mounted on the bone model (**b, d**), which helps find the right position when starting with the technique. A secure and unique fit can be demonstrated and verified

external rotation can be planned in this view. It is possible to change the external rotation reference from the epicondylar line to the posterior condyles or the Whiteside line. In the sagittal view, adjustment of the flexion/extension angle and the anterior/posterior position of the anterior cut is possible. The sagittal view includes a notch warning if the calculated exit of the saw blade does not exit the bone anteriorly and the notched area is larger than 1 mm^2.

A gap balancing feature gives an approximate estimation of the distance between the femoral distal cut plane and the tibial proximal cut plane in both flexion and extension. This provides additional information for the femoral and tibial resection, and thus a minimum resection depth is necessary to fit in the components depending on their thickness. Furthermore, it gives an idea of the required amount of mediolateral balancing of the flexion and extension gap.

The tibial planning consists of two 2D views, each aligned with one of the anatomical planes and the tibia anatomical axis. This results in a coronal and a sagittal view. In the coronal view, the distal resection depth and the varus/valgus angle can be adjusted. The sagittal view allows for planning of the posterior slope angle.

The 3D view displays the femur and tibia together or independently. The view can be rotated horizontally and vertically. It shows the implant with cut surfaces, the cut surfaces only, the implant covered by the bone without cut surfaces, or the bone model only with the landmarks.

In addition, this view allows for media/lateral placement of the femoral component when viewing the implant overlay.

A separate implant move mode for the tibia facilitates and improves the sizing, coverage, and rotation of the tibial component. Looking from above onto the semitransparent tibial component

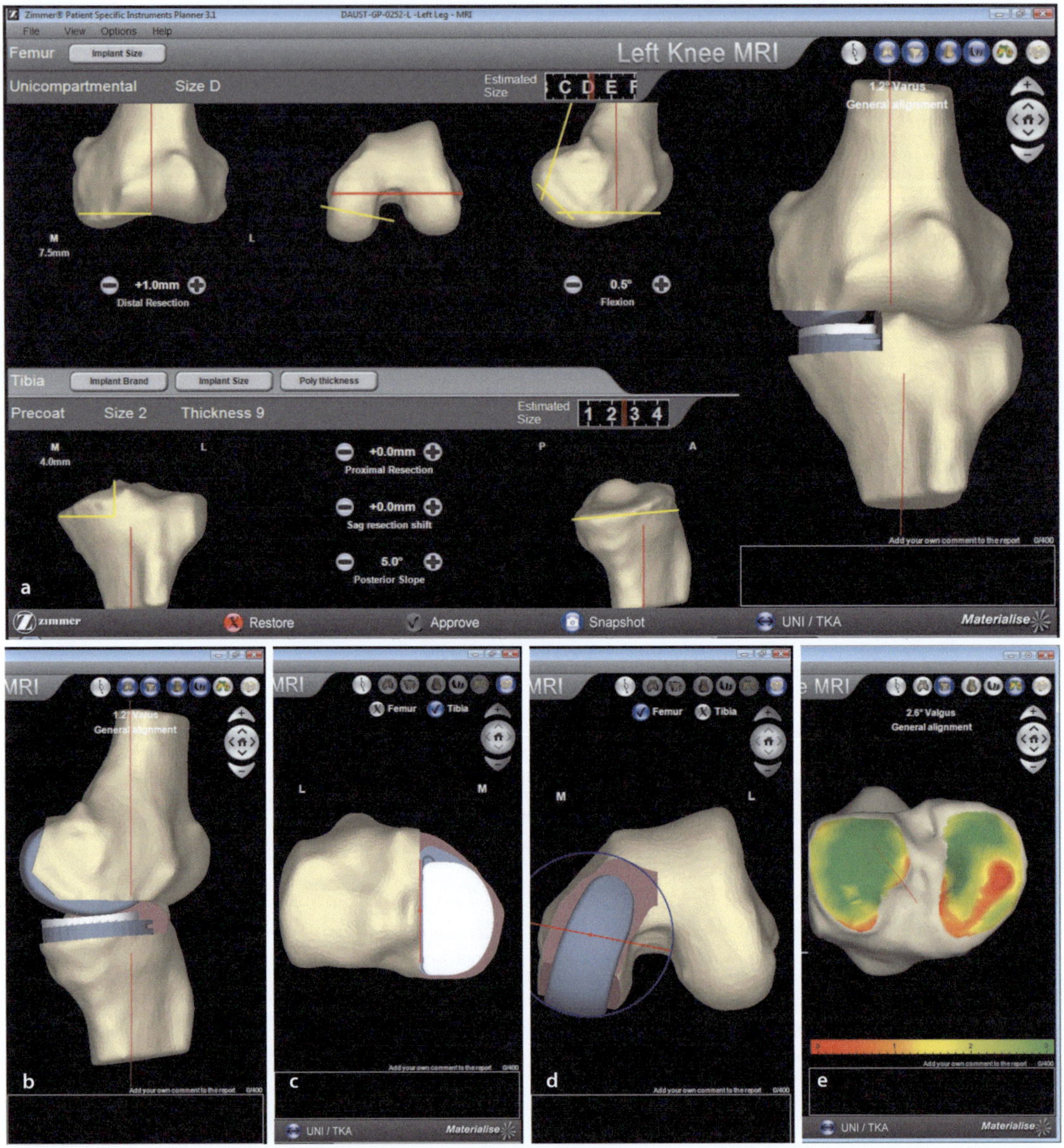

■ **Fig. 5.3a–e** The display for planning unicompartmental knee replacement (UNI) allows for modification of distal resection and flexion of the femoral component. For resection of the proximal tibial component, the sagittal resection shift and posterior slope can be changed (**a**). As in TKA, the orientation and sizing of the components can be controlled in the different 3D views (**b, c, d**). Cartilage mapping of the tibial side shows an anteromedial cartilage defect, which confirms the indication for UNI (**e**)

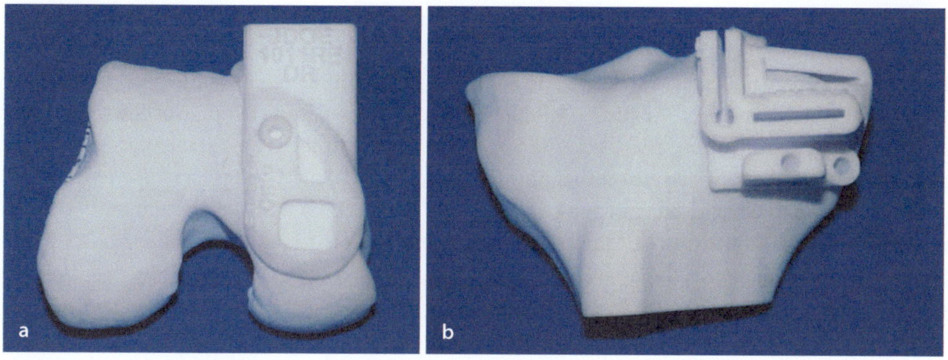

■ **Fig. 5.4a–b** Femoral (**a**) and tibial (**b**) cutting guide for unicompartmental replacement mounted on the bone model. Windows facilitate the verification of the bone contact

and the cut surface, the implant position can be changed in anterior/posterior and medial/lateral direction and it can be rotated. The overhang of the component is highlighted and can be detected.

After the planning is approved, 3D pin placement guides are designed using CAD software and subsequently manufactured (■ Fig. 5.2a–d).

5.5.2 Planning Unicompartmental Knee Replacement

The planning of UNI (■ Fig. 5.3a–e) is similar to that of TKA. For UNI, the estimated implant size is based on an anteroposterior measurement, which is made with the symmetry axis through the implant, keeping in mind that a gap of 2 mm should be present between the anterior border of the implant and the anterior border of the distal cutting plane.

In the coronal view of the femur, only the distal resection depth has to be evaluated; in the sagittal view, only the flexion/extension angle.

For the tibia, the size and thickness of the polyethylene can be chosen. The thickness of the polyethylene influences the varus/valgus angle that is indicated. Coronal and sagittal views of the tibia allow changes to be made in the proximal resection depth, in the sagittal resection shift, and in the posterior slope.

For UNI, the implant move mode is also available for the femoral component. The implant position can be adjusted by rotation and translation in a medial/lateral direction.

A cartilage color map represents the cartilage thickness reconstructed from MRI. The thickness and areal distribution of cartilage helps to verify the correct indication for the UNI. For each UNI case, the surgeon has the option of evaluating a preoperative TKA case as well.

3D cutting guides are produced for UNI (■ Fig. 5.4a,b).

5.6 Surgical Technique

5.6.1 Total Knee Replacement

The individual pin placement guides have to be sterilized in advance. The conventional instrument set for the chosen TKA can be used, and it can be reduced significantly since all the instruments for intra- and extramedullary alignment including the sizing guides are not needed.

The PSI technique can be employed with conventional and minimally invasive approaches. It is recommended to use it in conjunction with the femur-first technique.

After exposure of the knee, the femoral pin guide can be positioned. Osteophytes should not be removed because the shape of the pin guide is adapted to them and therefore they can be important for the correct placement of the instrument. The guide is captured by the anterior ridge of the femur. The epicondylar axis and anterior/posterior axis reference lines on the pin guide can be used to assess alignment. It may be helpful to apply the guide to the optionally included femoral bone model to check the correct position. By applying pressure to the guide in a posterior and lateral direction, a secure fit is achieved and the four pin holes can be drilled. After positioning the two anterior pins, the pin guide can be removed and the standard distal cutting block can be applied. The amount of medial and lateral resection can be estimated and, if useful, modified by changing the position of the cutting block proximally or distally by 2 or 4 mm. This can be the case if, for example, a relevant extension deficiency were to become obvious during examination of the knee under anesthesia. After the distal cut is performed, it can be helpful to replace the femoral pin guide in order to relocate the distal drill holes that are usually covered up by the cut. Using the guide, the distal pins can be placed and the 4-in-1 finishing guide can be applied. For correct placement, the medial/lateral position has to be adjusted as usual. The four cuts can be made after securing the cutting block and removing all pins (◘ Fig. 5.5a–c).

After removal of the menisci and the anterior cruciate ligament, the tibial pin guide can be positioned. This should be done without removing any osteophytes before for the same reason as in the femoral preparation. Proper placement of the tibial guide might require removal of soft tissue, in particular anteriorly. The posterior medial hook has to go over the posterior ridge of the tibia. The mechanical axis and proximal resection reference lines marked on the pin guide can be used to assess alignment. Like the femoral side, mounting the tibial guide on the bone model can help to find the correct position. The anterior lateral and medial pin holes can be drilled and pinned, while the two proximal pin holes will be drilled without placing the pins. The pin guide has to then be removed by lifting the medial hook. To do this without shifting the pins, it may be necessary to remove the anterior medial and occasionally also the anterior lateral pin, which have to be replaced to apply the tibial cutting guide. The alignment can be checked with the tibial alignment rod that should be parallel with respect to the tibial shaft. Resection depth and posterior slope can be assessed and modified as per the surgeon's discretion according to the conventional operative technique. After performing the proximal tibial cut, the tibial sizing plate can be put in place guided by the proximal pins that can be located in the drill holes using the tibial guide, if they are covered. Rotation and coverage of the tibial sizing plate can be modified at this stage. Among the different types of tibial plates, the selected one should be fixed and surgery can proceed following the standard operative technique (◘ Fig. 5.5d–f).

5.6.2 Unicompartmental Knee Replacement

The standard instrument set for the Zimmer® Unicompartmental High Flex Knee System can be reduced by removing the instruments for intra- and extramedullary alignment and the sizing guides and it must be complemented by the sterilized individual cutting guides. The UNI PSI technique can be performed with standard and minimally invasive approaches. Removal of the medial meniscus, at least anteriorly, should be performed in order to have exposure to the anterior portion of the medial plateau. Osteophytes should be left in place since the cutting guide is shaped according to the patient's bone and proper fit can rely on individual osteophytic formations. It might be necessary to remove some soft tissue for correct placement of the cutting guide. The guide is positioned on the medial tibial plateau by pressing it downward and posteriorly. A unique and stable fit must be verified as must contact with the bone. Contact can be checked through two windows and around the contact surface of the guide. The cutting block is then fixed with two screws. An additional pin is placed through the hole in the sagittal cut slot. Alignment can be checked with a rod mounted onto the guide. It should be parallel with the tibial crest in the frontal plane. First the proximal cut and then the sagittal cut should be performed. Both cuts will be stopped by the pin in the cut slot. After removal of the screws, pin, and cutting block, it might be necessary to complete the cut (◘ Fig. 5.6a,b).

The femoral cutting guide is positioned on the medial femoral condyle with the knee in 45° flexion. A unique and stable fit has to be verified, as well as bone contact using the windows. In full extension after inserting a tension guide between the

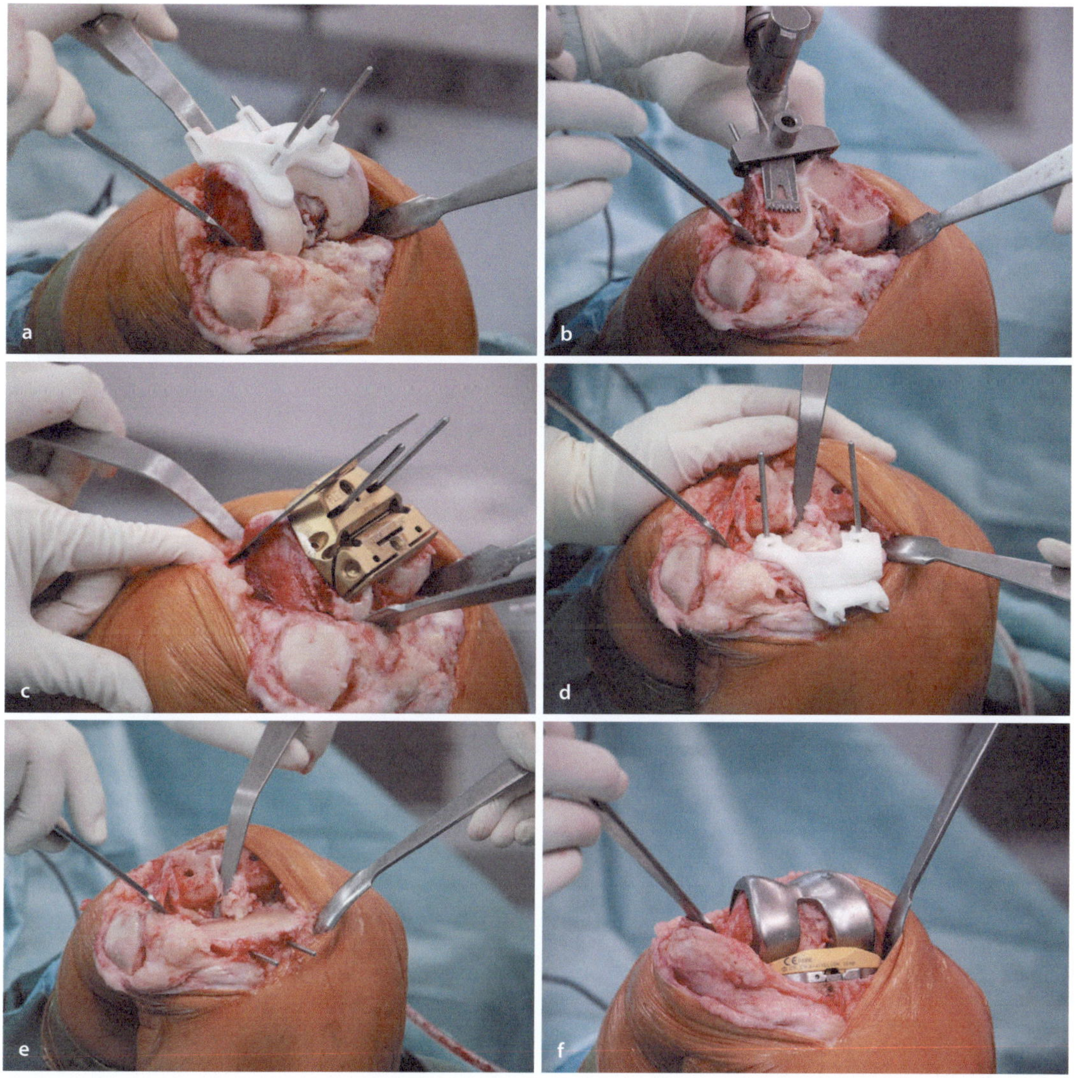

Fig. 5.5a–f The correct fit of the femoral (**a**) and tibial (**d**) pin guide in TKA is demonstrated intraoperatively. The anchored pins guide the standard instruments for the different cuts: distal femoral cutting instrument (**b**), 4-in-1 femoral cutting guide (**c**), and tibial resection (**e**). The trial implants demonstrate the correct size, orientation, and alignment (**f**)

femoral cutting block and the tibial cut, the cutting guide should be fixed by two screws. After removing the tension guide, the distal rotation pin cylinder can be drilled in slight flexion. In extension with the tension guide in place again, the distal femoral cut can then be performed. Subsequently, the cutting guide is removed and the femoral finishing guide of the planned size is placed and aligned over the predrilled hole and secured with a pin. Adjustment of femoral rotation can be made by rotating the finishing guide around this pin. The posterior surface of the femoral finishing guide should be parallel to the tibial cut. An underhang of 2–3 mm is visible when the component is sized properly. After fixation of the finishing guide, femoral preparation can be made according to the standard surgical technique. Overall alignment can be checked using a spacer block of the desired polyethylene thickness and the full-leg drop-down rod.

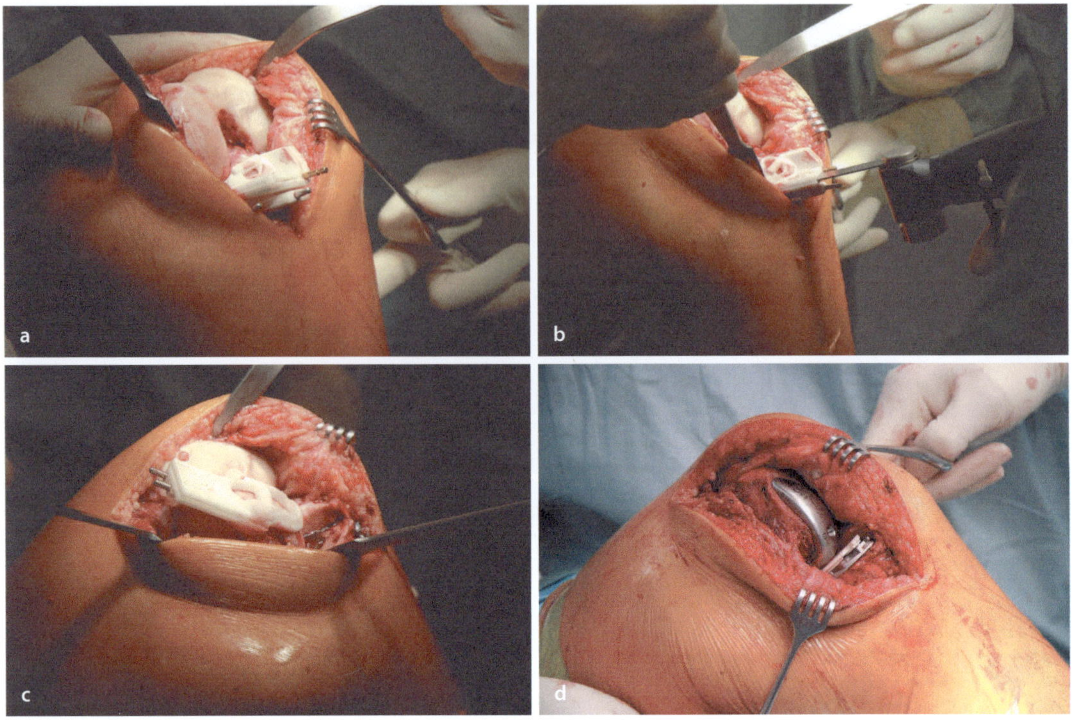

Fig. 5.6a–d In unicompartmental replacement, the cutting blocks are fixed on the tibial side first (**a**) followed by the tibial cuts (**b**). The femoral cutting block guides (**c**) the distal cut and placement of the finishing guide. Correct alignment and sizing of the UNI can be checked with the trial components (**d**)

If alignment is correct, the planned tibia size can be verified using the corresponding tibial spacer. The implantation is completed by following the standard surgical technique (Fig. 5.6c,d).

5.7 Initial Experience

At our institute, 32 total and 4 unicompartmental knee arthroplasties have been performed to date using the Zimmer® PSI technique. The patients suffered from disabling generalized primary osteoarthritis (TKA) or isolated medial osteoarthritis (UNI) with failed nonoperative treatment. The indications for PSI were the ability and willingness to undergo preoperative MRI and the acceptance of the relatively new technology. Exclusion criteria for PSI were metallic hardware within 150 mm of the knee. No other exclusion criteria were applied compared to conventionally operated patients.

In all selected patients, the MRI was performed according to the standard protocol. In three cases it had to be repeated because the patients changed position during the investigation resulting in motion artifacts. In four cases, the MRI revealed minor artifacts within 150 mm of the knee joint line, which could be neglected. In all cases, uploading of MRI images, preparing the files, segmentation, presurgical planning, designing, and manufacturing the guides as well as shipment were carried out in time and surgery could be performed as scheduled.

For all TKA cases, a Zimmer® NexGen CR-Flex fixed bearing knee system, and for all UNI cases the Zimmer® Unicompartmental High Flex Knee System could be planned appropriately and subsequently implanted. In certain cases, to support the indication for a unicompartmental replacement, cartilage mapping was used. In all the procedures, the pin placement guides and cutting guides had a stable and unique fit. Positioning of the tibial guides in TKA required more training when starting with

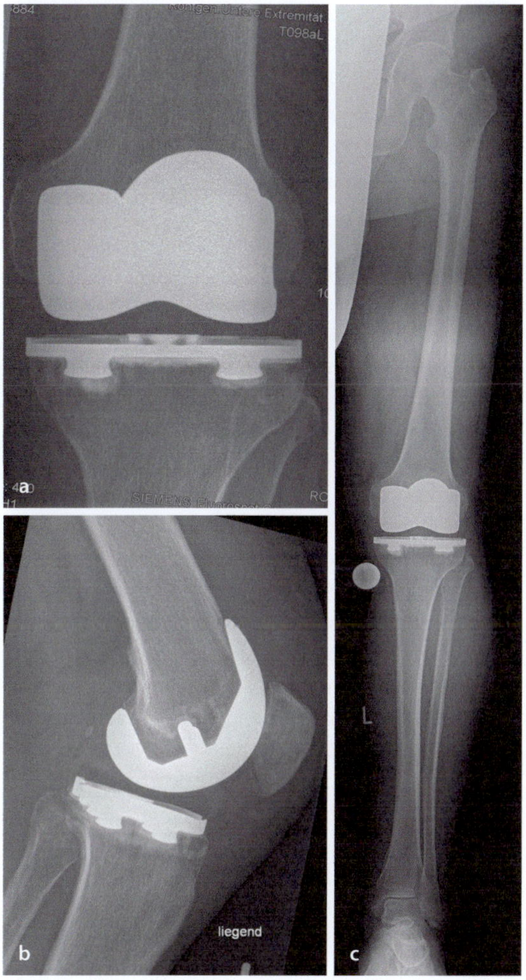

Fig. 5.7a–c Postoperative radiographs – anteroposterior (**a**), lateral (**b**), and anteroposterior (**c**) long-leg – of a TKA implanted using the PSI technique. The radiographs demonstrate the correct alignment

the system. Placing the guide on the tibia bone model before definitive in situ positioning was helpful in these cases. In one case, femoral rotation seemed to be too large and was checked using the standard instruments. Comparison of the two methods revealed no difference and surgery was completed using the PSI technique. In four cases, distal resection of the femur was carried out more proximally (3×2 mm, 1×4 mm) than planned because the extension deficiency of the knee was measured under anesthesia. A more distal tibial resection became necessary in five cases owing to a combined gap tightness in extension and flexion. Correction of tibial and femoral resection in this plane was needed less frequently after applying the gap balancing feature. In one case the tibial size had to be reduced intraoperatively in comparison to the preoperative planning. On the femoral side, no changes in varus/valgus orientation, extension/flexion, rotation (referenced to the epicondylar line), and anterior/posterior shifting became necessary. No femoral notching could be observed. During preparation of the tibia, the varus/valgus orientation and posterior slope were derived exactly without any divergence from the guides.

Intraoperative gap balancing could be performed according to the standard surgical technique without significant difficulties. No method-associated or general complication was observed intraoperatively.

Postoperative evaluation included measurement of the clinical and radiological outcome using our standard procedure. For clinical evaluation, the Oxford Knee Score, SF 12, UCLA Activity Score, and range of motion (ROM) were recorded. Radiological analysis was performed using standard anteroposterior and lateral as well as anteroposterior long-leg radiographs.

The outcome so far has revealed good clinical results. Joint stability was achieved in all cases. The minimum ROM at the time of discharge from hospital was at least 90°. Radiological results showed correct alignment in all cases. The overall mechanical axis (line between the center of the femoral head and the center of the proximal surface of the talar dome) passed through the central third of the knee in all cases. The overall hip–knee–ankle angle was always between 179°and 181° (±1°), the femoral and tibial component angle (angle between the femoral component and the femoral mechanical axis and between the tibial component and the tibial mechanical axis) was between 89° and 91° (Fig. 5.7a,b and Fig. 5.8a,b).

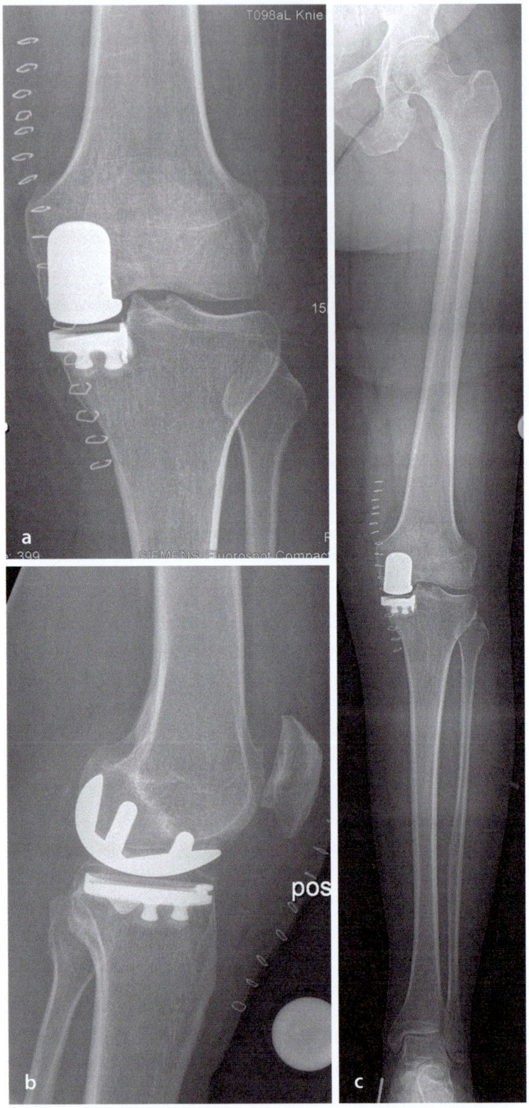

Fig. 5.8a–c Postoperative radiographs of UNI performed with PSI. The indented alignment has been achieved

5.8 Discussion

Patient-specific instrumentation using the PSI technology is based on the proven method of mechanical alignment in total and unicompartmental knee arthroplasty. Although alignment is not the only target and does not guarantee better clinical outcome and survivorship (Parratte et al. 2012; Matziolis et al. 2007), it has a significant influence on the results (Sikorski 2008). Neutral alignment is currently the subject of controversial discussion (Bellemans et al. 2012) and kinematic alignment (Dossett et al. 2012) is considered as an alternative procedure. Nevertheless, there is no evidence at present that alignment other than neutral should be recommended.

A remarkable advantage of the PSI technique is the ability to perform accurate preoperative planning, which refers to the bone resection and the type, size, and positioning of the implants. A selection of different implants, which have been proven in clinical practice over years, are available and can be adapted with respect to size, orientation, and variants to the individual anatomy. Our first experience has revealed that the surgical planning and technique are easy to handle and have a steep but short learning curve. Alignment could be achieved in the comparatively small group of patients using the available technology. However, further studies are necessary to compare alignment with the standard procedure and to assess patient satisfaction and functional outcome. As in other studies (Nunley et al. 2012; Watters et al. 2011), we have some evidence that operative time can be reduced with PSI as can the cost for processing the operative equipment.

Experience with PSI is still limited (Myer et al. 2012; Nunley et al. 2012a,b; Watters et al. 2011). When evaluating this new method it should be borne in mind that it is still in the early stages of development. Further development opportunities should be exploited before a final assessment is made. In particular, the current direct comparison with navigation makes little sense, since the latter has been developed over a period of more than 10 years. Possibly, a combination of the two methods is an option for the future. Disadvantages of navigation, such as the relatively high time-consuming procedure and the intra- and interindividual variations associated with the detection of landmarks and placement of the pins, could potentially be overcome. The current disadvantage of the PSI technique that intraoperative bone resection can be adapted to the soft tissue conditions only to a limited degree might be compensated for by complementary navigation steps in the future.

References

Bellemans J, Colyn W, Vandenneucker H, Victor J (2012) The Chitranjan Ranawat award: is neutral mechanical alignment normal for all patients? The concept of constitutional varus. Clin Orthop Relat Res 470:45–53

Chan KY, Teo YH (2012) Patient-specific instrumentation for total knee replacement verified by computer navigation: a case report. J Orthop Surg (Hong Kong) 20:111–114

Dossett HG, Swartz GJ, Estrada NA, Lefevre GW, Kwasman BG (2012) Kinematically versus mechanically aligned total knee arthroplasty. Orthopedics 35:160–169

Matziolis G, Krocker D, Weiss U, Tohtz S, Perka C (2007) A prospective, randomized study of computer-assisted and conventional total knee arthroplasty: three-dimensional evaluation of implant alignment and rotation. J Bone Joint Surg Am 89:236–243

Mayer SW, Hug KT, Hansen BJ, Bolognesi MP (2012) Total knee arthroplasty in osteopetrosis using patient-specific instrumentation. J Arthroplasty 27 [Epub ahead of print]

Ng VY, DeClaire JH, Berend KR, Gulick BC, Lombardi AV Jr. (2012) Improved accuracy of alignment with patient-specific positioning guides compared with manual instrumentation in TKA. Clin Orthop Relat Res 470:99–107

Nunley RM, Ellison BS, Zhu J, Ruh EL, Howell SM, Barrack RL (2012b) Do patient-specific guides improve coronal alignment in total knee arthroplasty? Clin Orthop Relat Res 470:895–902

Nunley RM, Ellison BS, Ruh EL, Williams BM, Foreman K, Ford AD, Barrack RL (2012a) Are patient-specific cutting blocks cost-effective for total knee arthroplasty? Clin Orthop Relat Res 470:889–894

Parratte S, Pagnano MW, Trousdale RT, Berry DJ (2010) Effect of postoperative mechanical axis alignment on the fifteen-year survival of modern, cemented total knee replacements. J Bone Joint Surg Am 92:2143–2149

Sikorski JM (2008) Alignment in total knee replacement. J Bone Joint Surg Br 90:1121–1127

Watters TS, Mather RC 3rd, Browne JA, Berend KR, Lombardi AV Jr, Bolognesi MP (2011) Analysis of procedure-related costs and proposed benefits of using patient-specific approach in total knee arthroplasty. J Surg Orthop Adv 20:112–116

The Individual-Template System Combined with Individual Endoprosthesis: ConforMIS™ iUni G2, iDuo G2, and iTotal G2

Andre F. Steinert, Ulrich Nöth, Maximilian Rudert

This chapter describes the basic rationale and surgical technique with uni-, bi-, or tricompartmental patient-specific knee arthroplasty using the second generation of ConforMIS™ implants. The patient-specific implants and instruments are designed and manufactured based on data from preoperative computed tomography (CT). The disposable patient-specific cutting jigs are fabricated with consideration of the anatomical and biomechanical axes of the knee, thereby resulting in efficient prenavigation of bony cuts without the need for an additional navigation system. For all types of resurfacing implants, the surgical technique comprises cartilage removal, knee balancing for determination of the optimal tibial resection, femoral and tibial preparation, trialing, and cementing of the implants. The use of personalized three-dimensional image-derived resurfacing implants, as well as individualized single-use instrumentation, has the potential to restore almost normal knee anatomy and kinematics and might therefore change the common surgical practice of knee arthroplasty.

6.1 Introduction to Individualized Knee Arthroplasty

The rationale of using patient-specific knee arthroplasty systems is based on the principle of fitting the knee implant to the patient's individual anatomy and pathology and not adjusting the patient's bony structures to the implant, which is the case in most standard knee replacement surgeries. The use of individualized implants and patient-specific cutting guides is thought to overcome some of the main problems of current standard knee arthroplasty such as abnormal knee kinematics, residual knee pain, reduced activity levels, and low patient satisfaction, among others (Banks et al. 2003; Bourne et al. 2010; Lezko et al. 2011; Noble et al. 2005).

The strive to generate individual knee arthroplasties was born from the observation that knee anatomy is strongly variable and that standard symmetrical knee implants cannot exactly restore the patient's knee surface morphology and natural knee kinematics in most of the cases, despite different sizes of implants being provided. Several anatomical and radiological studies show a high gender-specific variation in femur condyle sizes and radii from medial to lateral, including variability of the epicondylar axis, the trochlea surface morphology, and the tibia plateau geometry (Hernigou et al. 1991; Howell et al. 2010; Li et al. 2012; Luo et al. 2004; Tan et al. 2007). Moreover, there is also a very high interindividual variability of these structures, resulting in considerable differences in knee kinematics (Bellemans et al. 2005). Knee kinematics itself is very complex and the knee's motion sequence comprises a roll–slide mechanism during flexion and extension, including a final rotational movement at the end of the movement cycle (Flandry and Hommel 2011). Changes of the anatomical landmarks during knee arthroplasty are likely to result in changes of the interplay between the osseous and soft tissue structures involved, which may lead to pathologically altered knee kinematics (Fitzpatrick et al. 2012; Howell et al. 2012; Steinbruck et al. 2011). In this respect, current implant designs for partial and total knee replacement have several major limitations, as these implants do not resemble the patient's individual anatomy accurately, which results in associated problems. Examples of significant implant design flaws include: early failure rates of tibia plateaus of narrow total knee arthroplasty (TKA) designs in obese patients as compared to wider implant designs (Berend et al. 2005); mismatch of the tibial plateau with overhang or subsidence of the underlying bone; symmetric femoral components with increased edge-loading and subsequent component failure; or oversized femoral components resulting in patellofemoral impingement. Differences in the bony anatomy between male and female knees have been well documented, in that men have larger femurs than women (van den Heever et al. 2012). Although these characteristics have been addressed in the current gender-specific TKA designs on the market, several other interindividual differences including rotation differences of the trochlea relative to the epicondylar axis are not dealt with. Other TKA types were designed to change knee kinematics intentionally, such as single-radius implant designs for higher flexion performance (Borrione et al. 2011; Cook et al. 2012; Wolterbeek et al. 2012). However, such designs deal with altered knee kinematics and the potential risk for instability in deep flexion (Catani et al. 2011). In summary, individualized patient-specific implants can address the shortcomings of current off-the-shelf TKA implants and are able to increase osseous implant coverage. Therefore, this chapter presents and discusses a novel surgical technique that utilizes the second generation (G2) of patient-specific uni-, bi-, or tricompartmental resurfacing implants along with patient-specific personalized jigs for the treatment of different stages of osteoarthritis (OA).

6.2 Indications and Contraindications: Which Knee Implant for Which Patient?

The choice of which implant is best suited for the patient should always be an individual decision made by the patient together with their physician based on a rationale considering several factors including the extent and distribution of cartilage wear, underlying disease [OA, rheumatoid arthritis (RA) etc.], age, weight, activity level, and attitude toward potential revision surgery, among others. Therefore a thorough history of the patient's knee pain has to be taken, including evaluation for anterior knee pain, or nickel allergy, among others. Furthermore, a detailed physical examination is required that includes assessment of any knee ligament instability, patella pain, or maltracking. The diagnostic work-up generally includes standard anterior–posterior (AP) and lateral radiographs of the knee, a skyline view of the patella, as well as full weight-bearing long-leg radiographs for assessment of the mechanical knee axis. When the decision for a knee replacement has been made, it should be initially determined whether a partial knee arthroplasty (PKA) or a TKA is most suited to treat the patients' knee pathology. Generally, PKAs are less invasive than TKA surgeries with faster initial recovery, and usually OA patients are selected who are under 60 years of age with stable knees and less than 10° axis deformity (varus, valgus, flexion contracture) (Pennington et al. 2003). Depending on whether a unicompartmental (medial or lateral) or a bicompartmental joint (medial and retropatellar, or lateral and retropatellar) disease is prevalent, a unicompartmental or bicompartmental PKA is chosen. In cases where the choice of the most suitable implant is not entirely clear, magnetic resonance imaging (MRI) of the knee joint might be a helpful additional diagnostic tool for decision making. In some radiology centers, CT scans with injection of intra-articular contrast agents can be alternatively employed.

Having determined the type of desired implant, usually the decision is made whether an individualized knee implant or a standard knee replacement system should be chosen. Currently, contraindications for individualized knee arthroplasty using the ConforMIS™ system are infection, medial or lateral knee instability, insufficiency of the anterior cruciate ligament (iUni/iDuo) or posterior cruciate ligament (iTotal), >15° axis deformity (iTotal), and >10° fixed varus/valgus deformity (iUni/iDuo). Relative contraindications for partial knee replacements include RA, tricompartmental OA, and a body mass index of over 35.

Once patient and surgeon decide for individualized knee replacement surgery, an x-ray CT scan of the knee is performed for the design and fabrication of patient-specific implants and instruments, with the whole process taking 6 weeks until the implantation kit is delivered (Fig. 6.1).

6.3 Preoperative Planning and iView® Technology

The ConforMIS™ image-to-implant technology is based on the fabrication of patient-specific knee implants and instruments on the basis of CT images, with additional radiation exposure. Along with instruments and implants, prenavigational patient-specific iView® planning images are provided for all types of implants, including unicompartmental (Fig. 6.2a; iUni® G2), bicompartmental (Fig. 6.2b; iDuo® G2), or tricompartmental (Fig. 6.2c; iTotal® G2) knee resurfacing systems. For the unicompartmental (Fig. 6.2a; iUni® G2) knee replacement systems, iView images indicate any osteophytes in green and red, with the red osteophytes marking osteophytes that must be removed for correct positioning of the iJig® patient-specific instrumentation (Fig. 6.2a, left images). Additionally, information on the requested posterior condyle cut, tibial cut slope, and anterior cortex cut is provided, as well as the projected positioning

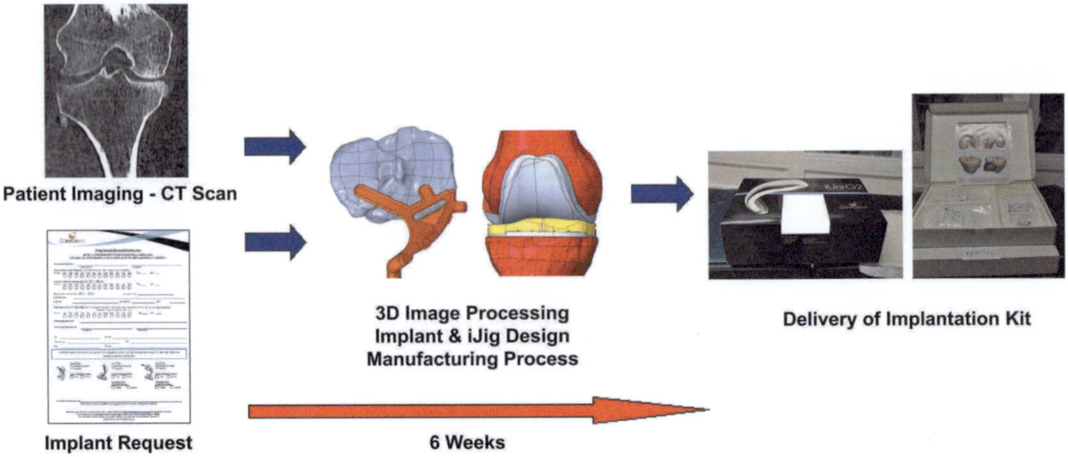

Fig. 6.1 Patient-specific knee arthroplasty organizational diagram. Once patient and surgeon have agreed to a patient-specific knee arthroplasty, the patient is referred to the radiology department for a CT scan of the knee to be treated, and the surgeon sends an implant request form to ConforMIS™, indicating patient data, implant requested, and scheduled surgery date. Upon receipt of the CT scan, images are processed and individualized implants and instruments are designed and fabricated within a 6-week timeframe. Implants and instruments are delivered thereafter in a convenient implantation kit (»lunchbox«)

implants for the femur and tibia (Fig. 6.2a). Similarly, iView images for the bicompartmental knee resurfacing system (Fig. 6.2b; iDuo® G2) indicate any disturbing osteophytes in red (Fig. 6.2b, left images), correct positioning of the femoral and tibial iJig® patient-specific cutting guides, data on the desired posterior condylar cut, tibial cut slope, and anterior cortex cut, as well as the targeted femoral and tibial implant positioning (Fig. 6.2b). The second generation of iView® (2.0) for the iTotal® G2 (Fig. 6.2c) indicates tibial and femoral positioning of the iJig® cutting blocks, proposed distal and AP femoral cuts, proposed tibial bone resection and slope, as well as projected femoral and tibial implant positioning (Fig. 6.2c). Notably, this prenavigation system allows for additional intraoperative confirmation of the projected bone cuts and facilitation of correct positioning of iUni® G2, iDuo® G2, or iTotal® G2 implants. The respective surgical techniques are outlined in the following paragraphs.

6.4 Individual Unicompartmental Knee Arthroplasty: iUni® G2

A major reason why unicompartmental knee arthroplasty is used in only a small percentage of patients with unicompartmental knee OA is that it is technically more demanding than TKA, with a surgical technique that is considered to be less reproducible (Fitz 2009). To overcome these limitations the iUni® G2 implant is designed for medial or lateral tibiofemoral compartment repair, using completely patient-specific implants and a set of patient-specific, disposable, and prenavigated cutting instruments (iJigs®; ConforMIS™). Design features of the iUni® G2 implant comprise an anatomically shaped femoral component that minimizes the need for bone removal and matching the anatomy of the tibial component for 100% cortical bone support that facilitates accurate fit. The iJigs are produced in such way that they fit the condyles in only one position that considers the biomechanical and anatomical axes from the CT scan, allowing for efficient prenavigation of cut planes without the need for a separate navigation system or an intramedullary alignment guide.

The surgical approach comprises a midline skin incision, a short medial (or lateral) parapatellar arthrotomy, and meniscus removal under protection of the collateral ligaments. The surgical technique includes the steps of cartilage and osteophyte removal, knee balancing, positioning of the tibial iJig®, tibial resection, positioning of the femoral

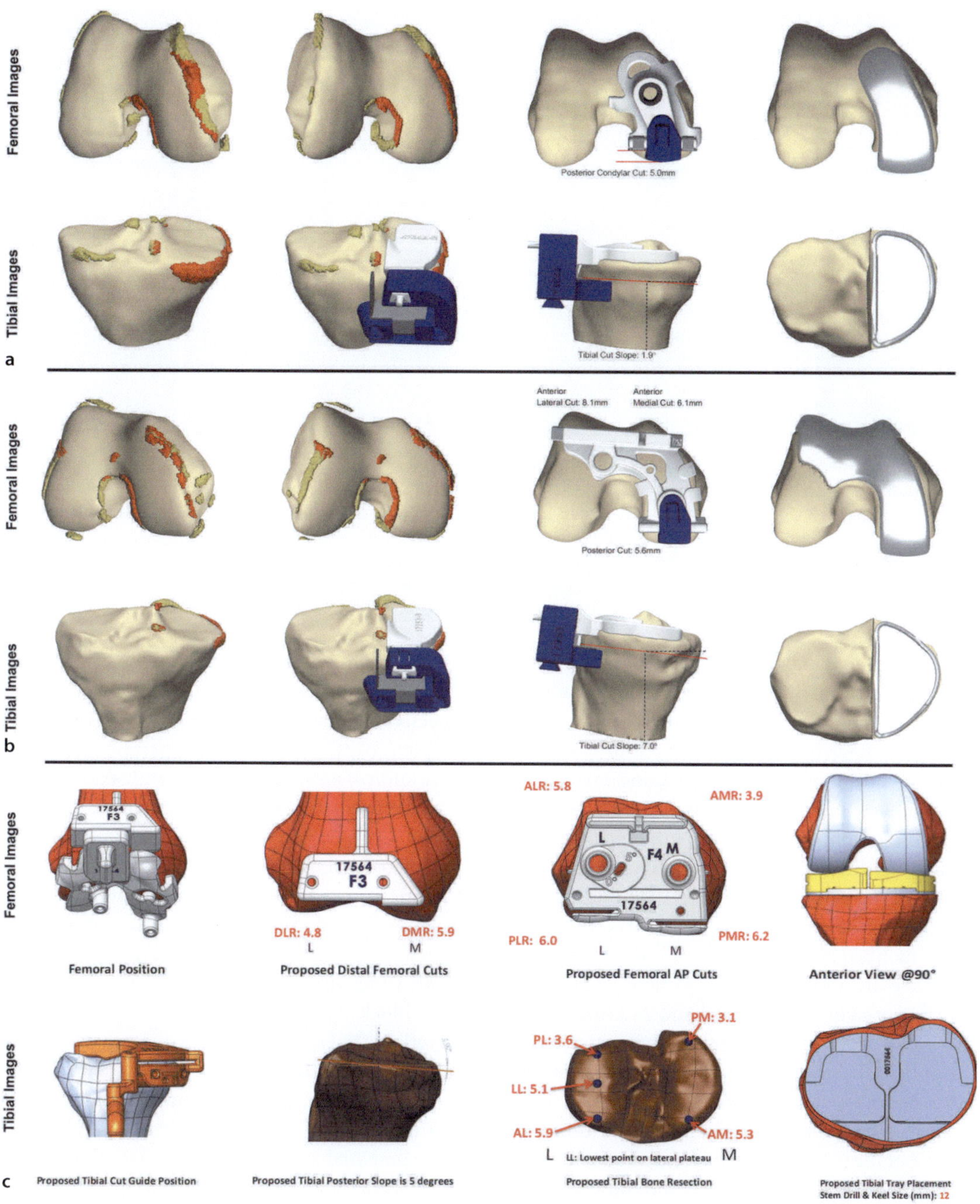

Fig. 6.2a–c Preoperative »navigation« using iView® patient-specific planning images. For all individual knee arthroplasties, iView patient-specific planning images are provided, indicating the positioning of cutting guides and implants for the femur and tibia (**a–c**). For the unicompartmental (**a**; iUni®) and the bicompartmental (**b**; iDuo®) knee replacement systems, iView images indicate any osteophytes in green and red, with the osteophytes in red indicating those that need to be removed for correct positioning of the iJig® patient-specific instrumentation. Additionally, information on the requested posterior condyle cut (**a, b**), tibial cut slope (**a, b**), and anterior cortex cut (**b**) is provided. **c** The iView 2.0 for the iTotal® G2 indicates tibial and femoral iJig® positioning, proposed distal and anteroposterior (*AP*) femoral cuts, proposed tibial bone resection and slope, as well as projected femoral and tibial implant positioning

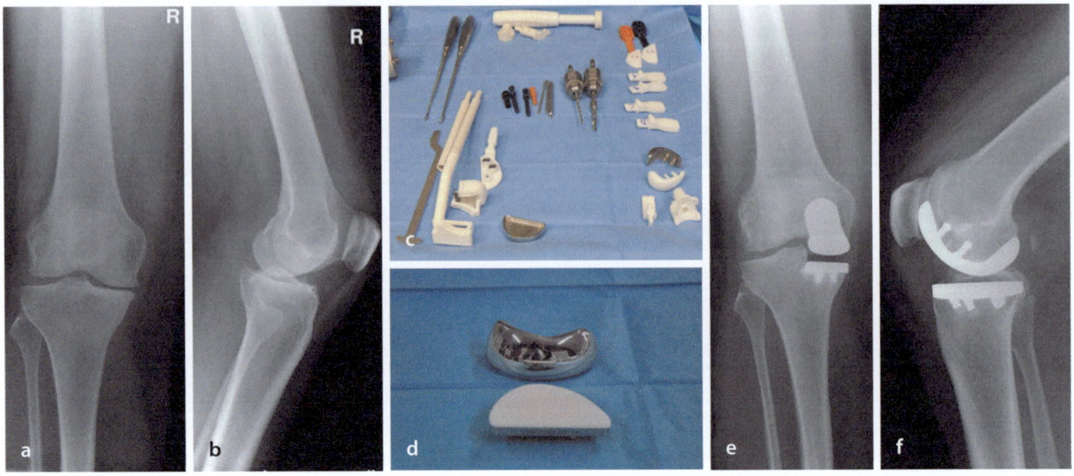

Fig. 6.3a–f Patient-specific unicondylar knee arthroplasty: ConforMIS™ iUni® G2. Preoperative AP (**a**) and lateral (**b**) radiographs indicate osteoarthritic changes in the medial compartment of the right knee of a 53-year-old female patient before medial iUni® G2 knee arthroplasty was scheduled. Examples of a patient-specific instrumentation kit including balancer chips, cutting guides, preparation set, and drill bits are depicted in **c**. An individual iUni® G2 implant is shown in **d** including a tibial component with a 6-mm polyethylene insert and a femoral component. Postoperative AP (**e**) and lateral (**f**) radiographs indicate correct implant positioning postoperatively without any implant overhang or subsidence (**e, f**)

iJig®, posterior condyle cut, final preparation of the femur and tibia, and final cementing of implants, as described in more detail elsewhere (Fitz 2009). Briefly, the linea terminalis of the femur is marked with the knee in extension, remaining cartilage in the compartment is removed with a curette, along with all osteophytes that might influence ligament tensioning and iJig® positioning. Balancer chips are then inserted in the compartment with 1-mm incremental thickness from A to D that exactly match the bony tibial surface, and knee laxity is tested in 20° knee flexion for ideal ligament tensioning, which is usually 1 mm medial and 2–3 mm lateral. The tibial iJig® cutting block is then attached to the optimal balancer chip (usually B or C) for performance of exact sagittal and horizontal tibial cuts, and an extramedullary rod allows for additional control of the varus/valgus axis and tibial slope. The bony tibial cut usually matches the individualized instrument for final tibial preparation exactly. Then, for femoral preparation, the knee is brought to 90° of flexion, and the femoral iJig® is correctly positioned to the femoral condyle, and subsequently drilled and pinned. Following this, an L-guide is attached to the femoral iJig® that represents the amount of bone to be removed and facilitates ideal posterior condyle resection, which is usually 3–5 mm including saw blade, as indicated in the respective iView® planning images (Fig. 6.2a). Completion of the femoral preparation includes preparation of an anterior groove with a 5-mm burr for the anterior corner of the femoral component that usually submerges the subchondral bone by 3.5 mm, as well as placement of 10–13 drill holes of 2 mm for improved cement interdigitation. Then the femoral trial component is inserted and the balancing is verified throughout the range of motion (ROM) using an 8-mm (orange) or a 10-mm tibial spacer block (blue) to prevent tightness and overcorrection (Fig. 6.3c). The 8-mm spacer block corresponds to the 6-mm polyethylene insert together with the 2-mm tibial tray. When no more bony resection is necessary, the tibial plateau is finally prepared with a tibial template that covers the tibial cortex and facilitates drilling of two holes and deepening of an inset with a chisel for the cementation peg of the tibial component. Then the original tibial tray and femoral trial components are used to verify the final implant fit and insert size, before the original components are implanted. Therefore, the tibial component is cemented first, then the original inlay is inserted and the femoral component is cemented, before all excess cement is removed and the knee is brought into 45° of flexion for cement hardening. Thereafter, closure of the arthrotomy and wound is performed in a standard fashion. Postoperative x-rays indicate the correct positioning of the final implant (◘ Fig. 6.3e,f).

6.5 Individual Bicompartmental Knee Arthroplasty: iDuo® G2

The clinical impact of degenerative changes of the patellofemoral joint in uni- and bicompartmental knee OA is controversially discussed (Breeman et al. 2011). In cases where a patellofemoral joint pain is clinically evident in bicompartmental OA, a bicompartmental knee resurfacing might be considered advantageous (Tria 2010). In this context, patients with one intact tibiofemoral knee compartment might be good candidates for treatment with a patient-specific bicompartmental knee arthroplasty-type ConforMIS™ iDuo G2. Such an approach has the advantage of resurfacing large areas of cartilage degeneration, while retaining the cruciate ligaments and therefore allowing for more normal knee kinematics. To close the gap between unicondylar knee arthroplasties and TKA in the care of bicompartmental OA, the iDuo® G2 implant is designed for medial or lateral tibiofemoral and retropatellar compartment repair, using individualized Jigs® and implants. Design features of the iDuo® G2 implant comprise a precise anatomical fit to ensure ROM without impingement or overhang, complete cortical rim coverage to avoid tibial component loosening or subsidence, and an anatomically shaped femoral component for maximum bone preservation. Similar to the iUni G2®, the iJigs® for the iDuo® G2 are manufactured such that they fit the condyles in only one position, facilitating efficient prenavigation of cut planes with consideration of the mechanical knee axis.

As mentioned previously for the iUni® G2, the surgical technique for the iDuo® G2 comprises a midline skin incision, parapatellar arthrotomy, meniscus and osteophyte removal, cartilage removal in the areas designated in the accompanying iView®, balancing the knee, positioning of tibial iJig® and tibial resection, positioning of the femorotrochlear iJig® and anterior and posterior condyle cut, final preparation of femur and tibia, and final cementing of the implants. In cases where patella resurfacing is intended, a spherical dome polyethylene patella implantation kit is provided.

The surgical steps include, briefly, marking of the linea terminalis of the femur along with the area of cartilage removal according to the iView® planning images. Cartilage remains in this area are removed with scalpel and curette, as well as all interfering osteophytes for iJig® positioning. Following knee balancing using incrementally sized balancing chips (A–D), the tibial iJig® cutting guide is fixed to the ideal balancer chip for accurate tibial bone cuts, with resected bone matching the tibial preparation guide exactly for confirmation. Then, the femoral iJig® is correctly placed to the femoral condyle and trochlea, and subsequently drilled and pinned, before the anterior and posterior femoral bone cuts are performed as planned in the respective iView® (◘ Fig. 6.2b). Femoral preparation is completed by preparing an anterior deepening recess of 3–4 mm, smoothening of bony edges, and placing several drill holes for cement interdigitation. Subsequently, the femoral trial component is inserted and the correct knee balancing is verified using the 8- or 10-mm spacer blocks. Final tibial preparation comprises drilling and preparation of a deepening for the pegs of the tibial tray, using the anatomical tibial preparation guide. The trial femur component, the trial inserts, and the original tibial tray are used to verify implant fit and insert choice, before the final components are implanted. Cementation is usually performed for the tibial plateau first, followed by the insertion of the final tibial plateau and cementation of the femoral component, using standard techniques. Following cement polymerization in 45° of knee flexion, the arthrotomy and wound are sutured closed using standard techniques. Postoperative x-rays indicate the accurate positioning of the final components with correct patella tracking (◘ Fig. 6.4e–g).

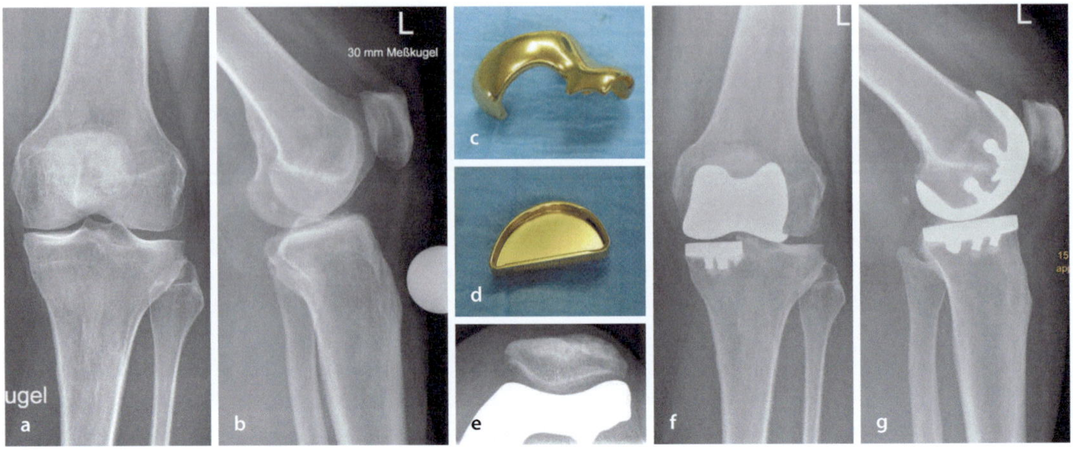

Fig. 6.4a–g Patient-specific bicondylar knee arthroplasty: ConforMIS™ iDuo® G2. Preoperative AP (**a**) and lateral (**b**) radiographs indicate osteoarthritic changes in the medial and to some extent in the retropatellar compartment of the left knee of a 56-year-old female patient, before medial and retropatellar iDuo® G2 knee resurfacing was scheduled. As this patient had a nickel allergy, the implant was surface-coated with titanium-nitride (TiN) hard coatings preoperatively, accounting for the »golden« appearance of the femoral (**c**) and TIBIAL component (**d**) before implantation. **e** Skyline-view radiographs of the patella indicate correct patella tracking postoperatively. Postoperative AP (**f**) and lateral (**g**) radiographs indicate correct implant positioning and cementation postoperatively without implant overhang or subsidence (**f, g**)

6.6 Individual Tricompartmental Knee Arthroplasty: iTotal® G2

Once tricompartmental OA is diagnosed and conservative treatment options fail, TKA surgery is usually offered. Although standard TKA survivorship is excellent, it has recently become apparent that patient satisfaction is not as good as we thought it was (Bourne et al. 2010). The reasons for dissatisfaction with standard TKA are very diverse and range from early implant failures due to leg misalignment, polyethylene wear, or engineering flaws, residual pain due to inappropriate component size and fit, malrotation of components, and functional compromises due to decreased range of motion, maltracking of the patella, or ligamentous imbalance that results in abnormal knee kinematics (Bonnin et al. 2010; Wylde et al. 2007). Recent surveys indicate that one in five patients is not satisfied with their TKA surgery (Bourne et al. 2006). To overcome these limitations, patient-specific iTotal® G2 was designed to fit exactly the patient's anatomy, in that the femoral component is shaped like the patient's knee restoring the patient's natural condylar curves (J-curves) from the medial to the lateral side. The tibial component matches the tibial plateau size exactly, as well as the femoral component, along with individual condylar spacing using different tibial plateaus medially and laterally, reduced resection of bone, and maximum coverage of the cortical bone resulting in large contact areas and low contact stresses (www.conformis.com). The surgical steps for performing iTotal® G2 consist in distal femoral resection, tibial resection, balancing and femoral preparation, tibial preparation, and final implant positioning. Patella resurfacing is also possible using oval dome-shaped polyethylene patellae of different sizes.

The surgical procedure is facilitated by using seven different patient-specific femoral and four different tibial instruments, which can be seen in Fig. 6.5c. First, the femoral block F1 is fitted onto the femoral condyles without the need for osteophyte removal, and cartilage is removed only at sites where the bony-referenced F2 and F3 blocks for the distal femoral cut are fixed. The distal cut is performed with the F3 block and usually creates an offset of the medial compared to the lateral condyle, mirroring the different condyle sizes. Then tibial cartilage is removed in areas where the bony-

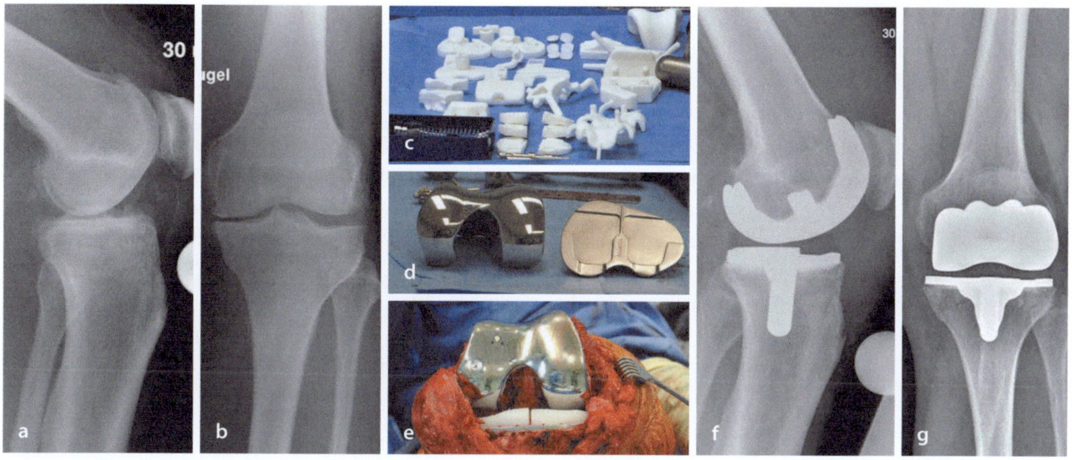

◘ **Fig. 6.5 Patient-specific total knee arthroplasty: ConforMIS™ iTotal® G2.** Preoperative lateral (**a**) and AP (**b**) radiographs indicate osteoarthritic changes in all compartments of the left knee of a 58-year-old male patient, before iTotal® G2 knee arthroplasty was scheduled. The patient-specific instrumentation kit including cutting and spacer blocks as well as trial components is shown in **c**. The individual iTotal® G2 femoral and tibial implant components before implantation are depicted in **d**. After implantation, these components reveal exact fit and alignment, with a 6-mm insert being implanted medially and a type A insert laterally (**e**). Postoperative lateral (**f**) and AP (**g**) radiographs indicate correct implant positioning postoperatively without any implant overhang or subsidence (**f, g**)

referenced T1 extramedullary cutting guide is positioned, as indicated in the respective iView® image (◘ Fig. 6.2c). Following alignment with a rod and fixation of the tibial cutting guide, the cut of the tibial plateau is made according to the iView® (◘ Fig. 6.2c). Then, the knee is balanced in extension with spacer block T2 and in flexion with spacer block T3. If tight, the system allows for an additional resection of 2 mm on the femur or tibia. With the knee in 90° flexion, the femoral cutting block F4 is placed on the femur, and up to 5° external rotation can be added to balance the flexion gap. Then the anterior and posterior cuts, the anterior chamfer cut, and drilling of lug holes are performed using F4. Two additional chamfer cuts for bone preservation are made next using the blocks F5 and F6. The tibial (T4) and femoral (F7) trials are then inserted and balancing throughout ROM is confirmed. T4 exists in two different heights, accounting for different insert options. The tibial trial (T4) fits anatomically to the tibial plateau, and allows for 5° of rotational variation. Once the final position of the tibial plateau is determined, the drill tower and keel punch are used for preparation before the final implant choices are cemented and inserted. The macroscopic appearance of a patient-specific iTotal® G2 implant before (◘ Fig. 6.5d) and after implantation (◘ Fig. 6.5e) is presented in Fig. 6.5. Postoperative x-rays indicate the accurate positioning of the final components (◘ Fig. 6.5f–g).

6.7 Summary and Perspectives

In summary, the introduction of patient-specific image-derived resurfacing implants as well as personalized single-use instrumentation has the potential to alter the current surgical practice for knee arthroplasty. The novel prenavigated ConforMIS™ technology requires an additional CT scan, which facilitates the design and fabrication of patient-specific knee implants for treatment of uni-, bi- or tricompartmental knee OA. Disadvantages of this implant system are a manufacturing time of 6 weeks, the increased costs for the implant, and that at present strong deformities (>15°) and instabilities cannot be treated with such implants. However, these developments are underway and might enter the market soon. The current implant design is completely novel, as it grossly resembles the patient's anatomy for all implant types (iUni® G2, iDuo® G2, iTotal® G2), aiming to preserve natural knee kinematics. Additional advantages are the femoral bone-preservation with enhanced cortical bone support of the tibia, overcoming critical design limitations of commercial off-the-shelf implants. However, the accuracy of the prenavigated jigs remains to be determined, and the long-term clinical outcomes compared to standard TKA with or without navigation or gap balancing still need to be established.

References

Banks SA, Harman MK, Bellemans J, Hodge WA (2003) Making sense of knee arthroplasty kinematics: news you can use. J Bone Joint Surg Am 85-A [Suppl 4]:64–72

Bellemans J, Robijns F, Duerinckx J, Banks S, Vandenneucker H (2005) The influence of tibial slope on maximal flexion after total knee arthroplasty. Knee Surg Sports Traumatol Arthrosc 13:193–196

Berend KR, Lombardi AV Jr, Mallory TH, Adams JB, Groseth KL (2005) Early failure of minimally invasive unicompartmental knee arthroplasty is associated with obesity. Clin Orthop Relat Res 440:60–66

Bonnin MP, Basiglini L, Archbold HA (2011) What are the factors of residual pain after uncomplicated TKA? Knee Surg Sports Traumatol Arthrosc 19:1411–1417

Borrione F, Bonnevialle P, Mabit C et al (2011) Scorpio single radius total knee arthroplasty. A minimal five-year follow-up multicentric study. Int Orthop 35:1777–1782

Bourne RB, Chesworth BM, Davis AM, Mahomed NN, Charron KD (2010) Patient satisfaction after total knee arthroplasty: who is satisfied and who is not? Clin Orthop Relat Res 468:57–63

Breeman S, Campbell M, Dakin H et al (2011) Patellar resurfacing in total knee replacement: five-year clinical and economic results of a large randomized controlled trial. J Bone Joint Surg Am 93:1473–1481

Catani F, Belvedere C, Ensini A, Feliciangeli A, Giannini S, Leardini A (2011) In-vivo knee kinematics in rotationally unconstrained total knee arthroplasty. J Orthop Res 29:1484–1490

Cook LE, Klika AK, Szubski CR, Rosneck J, Molloy R, Barsoum WK (2012) Functional outcomes used to compare single radius and multiradius of curvature designs in total knee arthroplasty. J Knee Surg 25:249–253

Fitz W (2009) Unicompartmental knee arthroplasty with use of novel patient-specific resurfacing implants and personalized jigs. J Bone Joint Surg Am 91 [Suppl 1]:69–76

Fitzpatrick CK, Clary CW, Rullkoetter PJ (2012) The role of patient, surgical, and implant design variation in total knee replacement performance. J Biomech 45:2092–2102

Flandry F, Hommel G (2011) Normal anatomy and biomechanics of the knee. Sports Med Arthrosc 19:82–92

Hernigou P, de Ladoucette A, Kooli M, Goutallier D (1991) [Anatomy of the trochleo-condylar junction and its consequences on the femoro-patellar joint in single-compartment prostheses]. Rev Chir Orthop Reparatrice Appar Mot 77:381–388

Howell SM, Chen J, Hull ML (2012) Variability of the location of the tibial tubercle affects the rotational alignment of the tibial component in kinematically aligned total knee arthroplasty. Knee Surg Sports Traumatol Arthrosc [Epub ahead of print]

Howell SM, Kuznik K, Hull ML, Siston RA (2010) Longitudinal shapes of the tibia and femur are unrelated and variable. Clin Orthop Relat Res 468:1142–1148

Leszko F, Hovinga KR, Lerner AL, Komistek RD, Mahfouz MR (2011) In vivo normal knee kinematics: is ethnicity or gender an influencing factor? Clin Orthop Relat Res 469:95–106

Li K, Langdale E, Tashman S, Harner C, Zhang X (2012) Gender and condylar differences in distal femur morphometry clarified by automated computer analyses. J Orthop Res 30:686–692

Luo CF, Zeng BF, Koshino T (2004) Transepicondylar line and condylar line as parameters for axial alignment in knee arthroplasty. Knee 11:213–217

Noble PC, Conditt MA, Cook KF, Mathis KB (2006) The John Insall Award: Patient expectations affect satisfaction with total knee arthroplasty. Clin Orthop Relat Res 452:35–43

Noble PC, Gordon MJ, Weiss JM, Reddix RN, Conditt MA, Mathis KB (2005) Does total knee replacement restore normal knee function? Clin Orthop Relat Res 431:157–165

Pennington DW, Swienckowski JJ, Lutes WB, Drake GN (2003) Unicompartmental knee arthroplasty in patients sixty years of age or younger. J Bone Joint Surg Am 85-A:1968–1973

Steinbruck A, Milz S, Woiczinski M et al (2011) Anatomy and biomechanics of the patellofemoral joint: physiological conditions and changes after total knee arthroplasty (in German). Orthopade 40:848–854

Tan CM, Liau JJ, Chen WT, Cheng CK (2007) The accuracy of posterior condylar angles measured by one MR image. Clin Orthop Relat Res 456:159–163

Tria AJ Jr (2010) Bicompartmental arthroplasty of the knee. Instr Course Lect 59:61–73

van den Heever DJ, Scheffer C, Erasmus P, Dillon E (2012) Classification of gender and race in the distal femur using self organising maps. Knee 19:488–492

Wolterbeek N, Garling EH, Mertens BJ, Nelissen RG, Valstar ER (2012) Kinematics and early migration in single-radius mobile- and fixed-bearing total knee prostheses. Clin Biomech (Bristol, Avon) 27:398–402

Wylde V, Dieppe P, Hewlett S, Learmonth ID (2007) Total knee replacement: is it really an effective procedure for all? Knee 14:417–423

Kinematic Alignment in Total Knee Arthroplasty with Stryker ShapeMatch® Technology

Tilman Calliess, Henning Windhagen

The Stryker ShapeMatch® Technology differs fundamentally to other templating concepts with respect to the alignment philosophy of the implant and the soft tissue management. The key principle of the ShapeMatch® Technology is to orientate the prosthetic components around the kinematic axes of the knee and thus to restore the physiological articular surface and the natural ligament isometry and motion of the knee. It is meant to improve rehabilitation, knee function, and patient satisfaction after total knee arthroplasty.

In previously introduced templating concepts, the placement of components is based on the widely accepted principle of classic mechanical alignment that considers the two-dimensional (2D) alignment of the limb and knee in the coronal or frontal plane. This requires the adjustment of a neutral hip–knee–ankle angle with proximal tibial and distal femoral joint line angles perpendicular to the mechanical axis and a rotational alignment set to bony landmarks. With the correction of congenital preoperative deformities, soft tissue balancing is necessary for achieving symmetric flexion and extension gaps and restoring motion and balance of the knee. In contrast to this, Stryker ShapeMatch® Technology aims for a three-dimensional (3D) kinematic alignment of the components whereby the femoral component is oriented to the axis about which the tibia flexes and extends. Likewise, the tibial component position is also oriented to the same transverse femoral axis so that the longitudinal axis of the tibia is perpendicular to the flexion–extension axis. In combination with a measured resection technique and a single-radius prosthesis design like the Stryker Triathlon®, the physiological articular surface is restored as is the physiological interrelationship of the kinematic axes. Stryker ShapeMatch® Technology uses proprietary software to estimate the patient's individual prearthritic condition so that the physiological joint line obliquity and the congenital overall limb alignment and rotation are preserved with the aim of restoring natural ligament isometry and motion of the knee.

This chapter reviews the definition and biomechanical rationale of kinematic alignment in total knee arthroplasty (TKA) and highlights the principle of the ShapeMatch® Technology to transfer the computed implant position to the operating room. The clinical application of this technique is described, from the indication and the preoperative planning to the surgical technique, including the specific balancing algorithm in kinematic alignment. Theoretical concerns of the technique are discussed along with the disadvantages of mechanical alignment, and finally preliminary clinical results of kinematically aligned TKA are reviewed.

7.1 Biomechanical Rationale of Kinematic Alignment

The biomechanical rationale for kinematic total knee alignment can be traced to classic research on the kinematics of the unloaded knee motion published by Hollister and coworkers (Hollister et al. 1993). Since the knee is a force-fit joint, the kinematics are defined by the relative relationship of the femur, patella, and tibia in motion and are determined by the joint surface and ligament structures. In this construct, three axes are specified governing the movement of the patella and tibia with respect to the femur. The primary axis is a transverse axis through the femur about which the tibia flexes and extends. Based on the assumption of a single-radius knee movement, it is defined by the center of a cylinder aligned to the articular surface of the femoral condyles (Fig. 7.1). The second axis describes the center of the patella movement and is again located transversely in the femur. It is strictly parallel to the before mentioned flexion–extension axis and projects proximally and anteriorly to the center of the condyles. The third axis is a longitudinal axis in the tibia about which internal and external rotation of the tibia occurs. This axis is set perpendicular to each of the two transverse axes in the femur (Fig. 7.1).

Although the three kinematic axes for knee motion have a clearly defined geometrical position and interrelationship to each other, they cannot be found during surgery by referencing bony landmarks or using 2D imaging studies. The classically used transepicondylar axis is only an approximation of the flexion–extension axis and involves a 2°–11° malalignment in the individual patient (Eckhoff

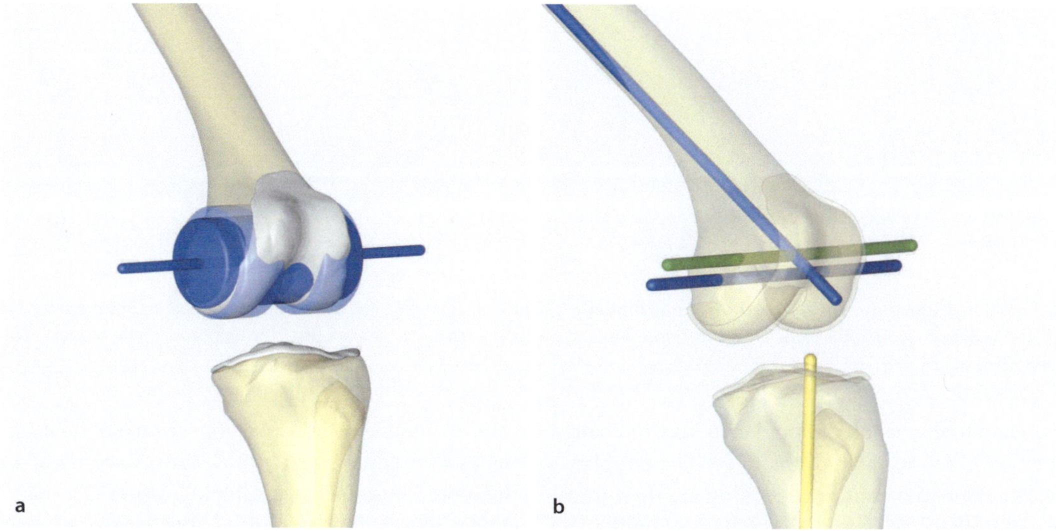

Fig. 7.1a,b Schema of the kinematic axes of the knee. a The primary transverse axis of the femur about which the tibia flexes and extends is defined by the center of a cylinder aligned to the articular surface of the femoral condyles. **b** The kinematic axis about which the patella flexes and extends is parallel to this and located anteriorly and proximally (*green*); the rotational axis of the tibia is perpendicular to each of the others (*yellow*)

et al. 2003). However, according to the geometrical definition, the primary flexion–extension axis of the femur can be calculated in a 3D model of knee, if the physiological prearthritic condition is restored, and hence the other two can be defined as well.

The design concept of kinematic total knee alignment is to coalign the femoral component to the primary transverse axis about which the tibia flexes and extends. Since this is a movement about a single radius and there is no clinically relevant asymmetry between the medial and lateral femoral condyles, a symmetrical single-radius femoral component is an optimal design for replicating knee kinematics. Hence, with a single-radius prosthesis it is as simple as shape matching the femoral component to the articular surface of the femur in a 3D prearthritic model. In the second step, the anterior–posterior axis of tibial component is aligned perpendicular to this now defined primary transverse femoral axis. The rotational alignment of the tibial component is set by marrying up the two restored bony models, such that the two deepest points of the femur sit in the sulci of the corresponding tibial articular surfaces, as would happen with load bearing. The femoral rotation is then projected onto the tibia. The final step is aligning the center of the tibia under the center of the prosthetic component.

7.2 Stryker ShapeMatch® Technology

The preoperative planning is performed on a 3D model of the patient's knee joint obtained from magnetic resonance images (MRI) or computed tomography arthrography (CT arthrography). For kinematic alignment, the projection of the knee has to be customized to the patient's knee position in the scanner so that the oblique sagittal image plane is perpendicular to the primary transverse axis of the femur. The crucial step for the calculation of the individual flexion–extension axis is transforming the arthritic knee model to the prearthritic status by filling articular defects and removing osteophytes (Fig. 7.2). This is done using proprietary software. By adjusting the varus–valgus rotation and proximal–distal position of the tibia, equal medial and lateral flexion and extension gaps are achieved and the physiological ligament length is restored.

The femoral and tibial components that best fit to this prearthritic knee are selected and shape

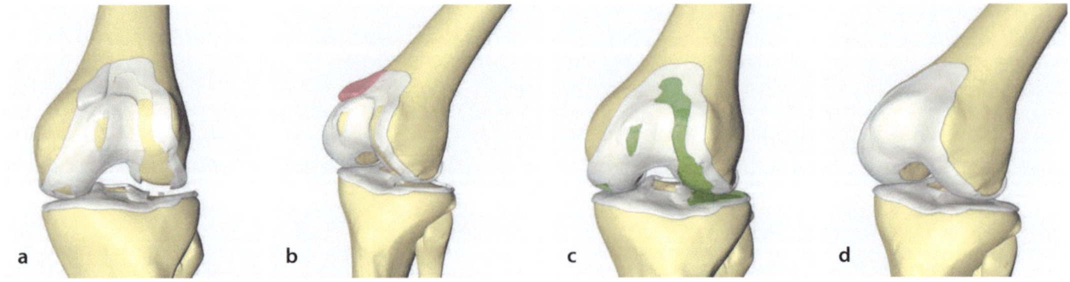

Fig. 7.2a–d Illustration of a 3D arthritic knee model. a The arthritic knee model; **b** with the process of removing osteophytes; **c** filling in worn joint surfaces; **d** centering the tibia under the femur to create a prearthritic normal knee model with the software

matched to the restored articular surface to coalign the above-defined axes of the knee. The cut planes for the defined component position are then transferred back to the arthritic model so that individual patient cutting guides can be machined to fit the actual arthritic patient's knee. Each template has three contact areas to the joint surface and sets the position of the component in the six possible degrees of freedom. The saw slots guide the proximal–distal, the flexion–extension, and the varus–valgus alignment of each femoral and tibial component, whereas the two pinholes on the articular surfaces of each cutting guide define the anterior–posterior (a.p.) and mediolateral (m.l.) position as well as the rotational alignment.

7.3 Clinical Application of Kinematically Aligned TKA

7.3.1 Indication

Since the primary goal of kinematic alignment in TKA is the preservation or restoration of the normal interrelationship among the kinematic axes of the prearthritic knee, this technique is applicable only for primary osteoarthritis. Posttraumatic conditions or a history of tibial or femoral correction osteotomies affecting the natural knee movement are, in the hands of the authors, contraindications for kinematic alignment. The same applies to soft tissue injuries or inflammatory arthritis affecting the primary ligament length and stability of the knee.

The overall varus or valgus alignment of the limb in the osteoarthritic condition does not represent an inclusion or exclusion criterion. The patient's individual prearthritic status is restored in the aforementioned planning algorithm. The physiological joint line obliquity in the coronal plane is preserved. This in turn means that a preexisting physiological varus or valgus deviation is accepted and left as it was.

The feasibility, safety, and tolerability of the kinematic approach are discussed in a separate section in this chapter. Admittedly, at present, with the current experience with this new technology and against the background of the current doctrine of a mechanical alignment of ±3°, the authors try to restrict the indications for kinematic alignment to patients whose physiological axis would meet the accepted range of deviation. In our preoperative algorithm the medial proximal tibial angle (MPTA) and the mechanical lateral distal femoral angle (mLDFA) are evaluated on long-leg standing radiographs and should be within the range of 85° to 90°. Additionally, the sum of the MPTA and the corresponding mechanical medial distal femoral angle (mMDFA) should be within 177°–183°. By this simple analysis the postoperative alignment and suitability for kinematic alignment can be estimated.

7.3.2 Preoperative Planning

Based on the preoperative imaging, an initial preoperative plan of the kinematic alignment is sent to the surgeon for approval. The planned implant position with regard to the coronal, sagittal, and axial plane is visualized on the basis of planning images (Fig. 7.3). The component sizes, together with the

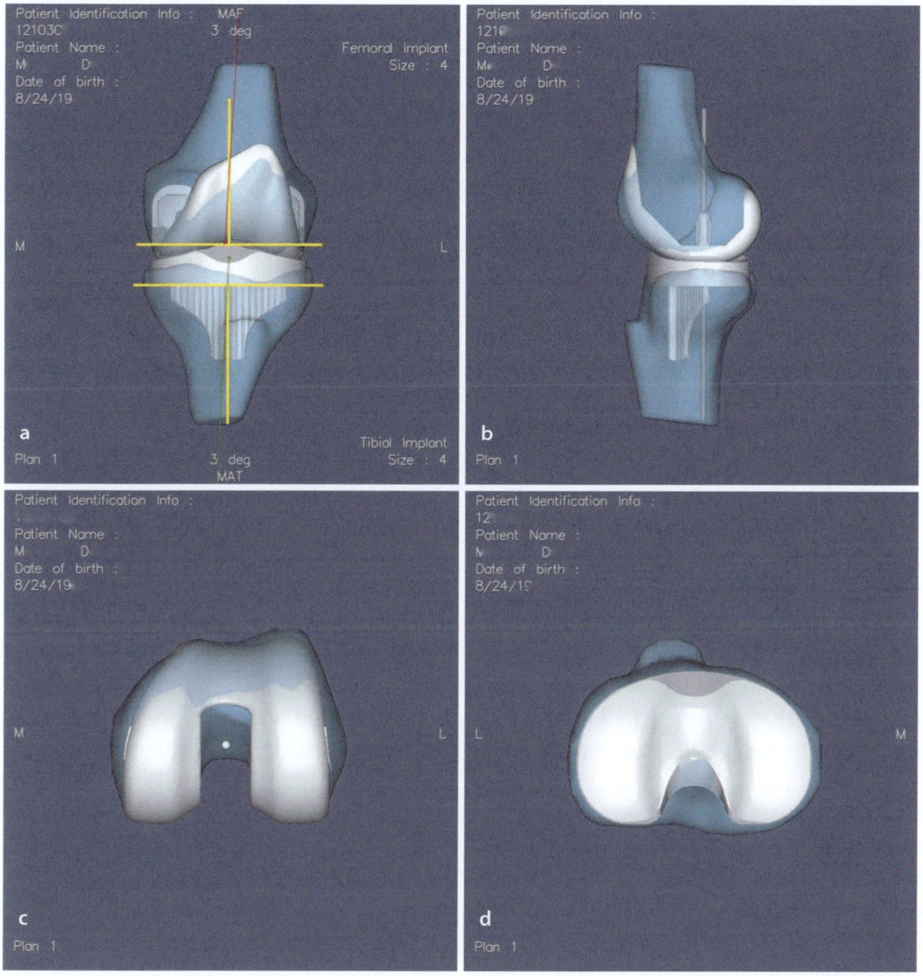

■ **Fig. 7.3a–d Illustration of preoperative planning sketches. a** Coronal, **b** sagittal, **c** axial femoral, and **d** tibial view. The medial proximal tibial angle, the mechanical lateral distal femoral angle, and the mechanical femoral and tibial axes are visualized in the coronal model along with the planned components

coronal alignment with regard to the joint line obliquity and the overall limb alignment, are specified. The tibial and femoral varus–valgus joint line angles and the overall femorotibial alignment parameters can be reviewed and accepted or modified as deemed appropriate by the prescribing surgeon. All the other parameters including component rotation, posterior tibial slope, bone cut thickness, or the component sizes are determined by the ShapeMatch® planning software. This approach appears appropriate for the complexity and the concept of kinematic alignment; however, the authors suggest that more parameters are visualized in the future so that the specified operation plan may be more traceable and better validated during the operative procedure.

In our algorithm the surgeon, on the basis of plane radiographs, validates the given preoperative plan. In case of a designated varus or valgus deviation of more than 3° from the mechanical axis or a joint line obliquity of more than 5° from 90, we currently tend to correct the tibial joint line angle until we meet the reference interval. The femoral alignment is never amended, as this defines the flexion–extension axis of the tibia and the patella tracking.

7.3.3 Operational Technique and Balancing Algorithm

The eventual surgical technique with the ShapeMatch® cutting guides does not significantly differ from that of other manufacturers and alignment concepts. The known advantages of a reduced number of instruments, decreased operating time, faster room turnover, and a simplified surgical procedure apply here as well.

The first difference to other systems is that, owing to the different planning algorithm and design of the ShapeMatch® guide, prominent osteophytes extending from the proximal trochlea or the notch are removed prior to seating the guide. In common with other systems, meticulous removal of soft tissue from the seating areas of the templates is mandatory.

Following removal of the distal bone using the position of the predetermined slot in the ShapeMatch® guide, the appropriate-size conventional 4-in-1 femoral block is inserted into the two articular pinholes that were used to secure the ShapeMatch® guide. On the tibial side, once again following predetermined proximal tibial resection, the two articular pins used to secure the template set the final position of the tibial trial. In our experience, small parallel adjustments of the a.p. or m.l. position may be required to center the tibial component.

A goniometer can be used to check the intraoperative application of the plan-i.e., if the plan had a tibial varus of 2, then the goniometer would read this when set to the ankle. The essential step for verification of the correct positioning of the templates is the evaluation of the thickness of resected bone fragments. Since kinematic alignment is a measured resection technique for restoring the articular surface, the two distal and two posterior femoral resections should be perfectly symmetrical after correcting for cartilage and bone wear. In an osteoarthritic knee, we typically observe a 2- to 1-mm cartilage wear on the affected side of the distal femur and occasionally additional bone wear, usually not more than 1 mm. For varus osteoarthritis, for example, this results in a distal medial resection thickness of 1–2 mm less than the lateral portion. Taking the saw blade thickness into account, the resection on the unaffected side would be 6.5-mm thick. The same applies for the posterior resection, which typically has a 1-mm cartilage wear. Measuring the definite resection levels during surgery using a caliper is suitable for assessing the correct position of the template (◘ Fig. 7.4).

A similar algorithm also applies for the tibial bone cut. The thickness of the worn side should be thinner than the unworn side according to the amount of wear. However, the use of a caliper is more difficult because of the concave and convex anatomy of the tibial plateau. The tibial slope is planned for neutral alignment, so that the posterior resection tends to be thinner or at least the same as the anterior one. The correct position of the template can be confirmed by replacing the resected plateau in the patient-specific cutting guide (◘ Fig. 7.4).

The concept of kinematically aligned TKA is based on the idea of restoring the natural length, tension, and motion of the ligaments. Thus, balancing techniques addressing the ligament structures are not indicated. By restoring the articular surface and interrelationship among the kinematic axes, the need for balancing should be reduced to a minimum. The first critical step is to remove any osteophytes that interfere with the ligament position. Secondly, the posterior capsule should be released in preoperative flexion contracture or intraoperative extension lack.

The only soft tissue release in our algorithm is that of iliotibial tract release in case of an existing long-term valgus osteoarthritis. If the posterior cruciate ligament (PCL) is insufficient and a.p. instability is present and cannot be corrected by using a thicker polyethylene insert, we would opt for a posterior-stabilized component. However, it must be clarified that the ShapeMatch® Technology, in principle, is most appropriately applied to cruciate-retaining Triathlon® components. Sacrificing the PCL means that a decisive connection between the tibia and femur is lost, which may result in an imbalance between the flexion and extension gap. Thus, the aspired perfect stability around the single radius of the femoral component achieved by simply restoring the physiological ligament length may be affected.

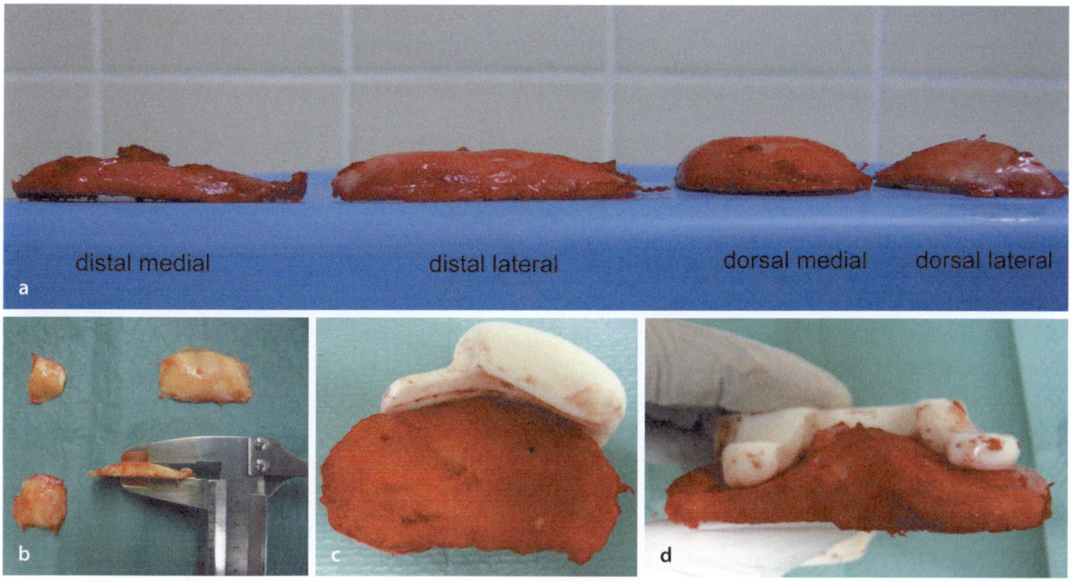

Fig. 7.4a–d Intraoperative confirmation of the correct kinematic alignment of the femoral component is made by measuring and comparing the symmetry of the thickness of the distal medial and lateral and posterior medial and lateral bone resections. **a** Typical example of varus gonarthrosis, with predominant medial distal wear. **b** Resection thickness is measured using a caliper. **c,d** Tibial resection is also reassured by placing the resected plateau into the patient-specific cutting guide

7.4 Controversy of Mechanical Versus Kinematic Alignment

Almost every study reviewing patient satisfaction and functional outcome after – mechanically aligned – TKA reports that about 20% of the patients are dissatisfied because of continued pain and poor function in activities of daily living (Baker et al. 2007; Bourne et al. 2010). Even the use of computer navigation resulting in a more accurate component alignment to the mechanical axis has not improved the clinical outcome (Cheng et al. 2012; Gothesen et al. 2011). On the contrary, data from the Scandinavian arthroplasty registries have shown that the risk of revision was even higher with the use of navigation (Gothesen et al. 2011).

Therefore, a mechanically aligned TKA has an unacceptably high prevalence of continued pain, poor function, and patient dissatisfaction. Moreover, studies have shown that the surgeon's intraoperative impression of the quality of the procedure, balance, and component position has no predictive value or correlation with the clinical outcome (Lee and Lotke 2012). This means that there is ample room for improvement in TKA, and there is reasonable doubt that this can be achieved with the use of conventional techniques and alignment philosophies. It is therefore dubious that other recently introduced templating concepts based on the idea of mechanical alignment would contribute to a better patient outcome.

The primary argument for mechanical alignment is that a neutral 0° hip–knee–ankle axis will result in better implant survivorship; however, the scientific support for this convention is surprisingly weak. Most of the literature reporting that prostheses positioned more than 3° deviant to the mechanical axis have a higher failure rate and higher risk of revision surgery dates back to the 1990s when very early knee designs and early generations of implant materials and instruments were used (Jeffery et al. 1991; Ritter et al. 1994). The more recent papers evaluating the survivorship of modern implant designs showed that factors other than alignment to the mechanical axis are more important for determining the survivorship at 15 years. On the basis of their evaluation, Paratte and coworkers stated in 2010 that the surgical goal of neutral hip–knee–

ankle alignment in TKA should be revisited (Parratte et al. 2010). This point is further raised with the findings of Magnussen and coworkers, who reported that patients with a preoperative varus deformity had the best outcome scores when left in a varus deformity after TKA (Magnussen et al. 2011). Even though the difference to neutral alignment was not significant, the inadvertently valgus-aligned knees did significantly worse.

Referencing the bone cuts to the femoral head and the center of the ankle in TKA changes the anatomical joint line of the femur and tibia in the axial and coronal plane and therefore results in kinematic malalignment of the knee. This may lead to ligament imbalance and explains the reported problem of midflexion instability. The same applies to the rotational alignment of the femur to the transepicondylar axis that may result in flexion instability especially in valgus knees with patella maltracking.

In kinematically aligned TKA, the individual patient's prearthritic varus or valgus deviation is restored and left as it was. However, on the basis of several studies, the average hip–knee–ankle axis is similar to that of conventional mechanical alignment (Spencer et al. 2009; Bellemans et al. 2012. Even though anatomical studies have shown that 98% of normal subjects do not have a neutral hip–knee–ankle axis, approximately 76% of the patients would be within a ±3° deviation (Bellemans et al. 2012). There are several case reports of successful kinematically aligned total knee replacements with a severe varus or valgus deviation in the short-term follow-up.

As early as 1988, John Insall reported in his paper on the *choices and compromises in total knee arthroplasty* that although there is consensus that the best alignment corresponds to the mechanical axis, this, in itself, is only a compromise (Insall 1988). He remarked that this position does not necessarily correspond to the original anatomy of the individual patient nor does it necessarily predict even loading across the prosthetic surface.

Kinematic alignment in TKA aims to restore the normal interrelationship of the kinematic axes and the physiological ligament tension and stability. We hypothesize that this could reduce the high prevalence of persistent pain and poor function in TKA.

7.5 Early Clinical Experience and Results

Stephen Howell, MD, Sacramento, completed the first kinematically aligned TKA using patient-specific cutting guides from OtisMed Corporation in January 2006. Stryker Corporation subsequently acquired OtisMed Corporation; in December 2010, Stryker SA Europe were granted market clearance by the European Competent Authorities to market and sell kinematically aligned ShapeMatch® cutting guides for use with the Triathlon® Total Knee System.

By the summer of 2012, the clinical experience of the European ShapeMatch® group comprised more than 500 kinematically aligned TKAs. The authors have contributed to this with approximately 50 patients, having completed our first ShapeMatch® procedure in October 2011. Today ShapeMatch® is part of our clinical routine for primary TKA for patients who meet the previously mentioned inclusion criteria.

In our series, all selected patients were within the given range of an overall limb alignment of ±3° to the mechanical axis in the preoperative planning, with the exception of three cases. In these cases the tibial varus angle was corrected until the overall limb alignment was acceptable. This involved a correction of about 2°–3° each and the resulting hip–knee–ankle angle was 3° of residual varus.

The ShapeMatch® cutting guides showed a good fit in all cases and there was no switch to the conventional instruments. The size of the planned femoral and tibial component matched the implanted size in every knee. As suggested by the theory, no soft tissue releases were necessary to achieve perfect stability and balance in any of the cases. The knee was balanced by removing marginal osteophytes, which indirectly lengthened the tight ligaments. In the cases for which we had made adjustments to the initial alignment proposal, the balancer tool used during surgery showed a symmetrical 2° misbalance over the motion arc; however, since overall stability was satisfactory no effort for correction was made.

The only soft tissue release conducted in our series addressed the iliotibial tract that appeared to be tight in two cases, both of which were patients who had a long-standing arthritic valgus deviation.

The PCL showed a perfect balance in all patients with a physiological roll-back motion in deep flexion and an a.p. shift of usually less than 0.5 cm. Only in one case of inadvertent injury of the PCL did we switch to a posterior-stabilized component.

The default preoperative plan aims for an 11-mm polyethylene insert; however, in about half of the cases a 9- or 13-mm polyethylene insert was used to achieve perfect stability and full range of motion. By using the ShapeMatch® cutting guides, the mean operating time was reduced to 45 min so that we were usually able to operate five to six knees a day, in contrast to our previous typical rate of four.

Although the overall evidence on kinematic alignment in TKA is still low, several studies utilizing the OtisMed Corporation product have described early clinical benefits in comparison to classic mechanical alignment (Dossett et al. 2012; Howell et al. 2008). Dossett and coworkers published a randomized, controlled trial of 41 kinematically aligned versus 41 mechanically aligned TKAs. They showed significant improvement in several outcome scores as well as a greater flexion (5.0°, p=0.043) in the kinematically aligned group 6 months postoperatively. However, the hip–knee–ankle angle (0.3° difference; p=0.693) and the anatomic angle of the knee (0.8° difference, p=0.131) were similar for both groups, and differences were identified for the joint line obliquity (p<0.000), which was suspected (Dossett et al. 2012).

The authors are currently taking part in two prospective studies comparing conventional instrumented TKA with the kinematically aligned ShapeMatch® Technology and also mechanically aligned cutting guides. One of these is a European prospective randomized controlled multicenter trial.

7.6 Summary

In summary, the Stryker ShapeMatch® patient-specific cutting guides are not about the templating technology itself, but are about realizing the kinematic alignment philosophy; in this concept the patient-specific guides are a necessary tool for transferring the computed 3D implant position to the operating room. The coalignment of the primary transverse flexion–extension axis of the femur to the single-radius axis of the prosthesis and the restoration of the natural ligament stability of the knee appear to be a logical step in improving the performance of primary TKA.

In our hands, the kinematic alignment philosophy realized with ShapeMatch® Technology is an evolution of the current mechanical alignment practice. However, long-term clinical benefit and implant longevity are yet to be proven. The suitability of kinematic alignment in severe varus or valgus deformities is also of special interest; currently, we correct these cases on the tibial side to an acceptable residual varus or valgus alignment of 3° to the mechanical axis.

There is a need for level-I studies to clarify the differences between mechanical and kinematic alignment with the use of patient-specific guides as well as to optimize the indications for both strategies.

References

Baker PN, van der Meulen JH, Lewsey J et al (2007) The role of pain and function in determining patient satisfaction after total knee replacement. Data from the National Joint Registry for England and Wales. J Bone Joint Surg Br 89:893–900

Bellemans J, Colyn W, Vandenneucker H et al (2012) The Chitranjan Ranawat award: is neutral mechanical alignment normal for all patients? The concept of constitutional varus. Clin Orthop Relat Res 470:45–53

Bourne RB, Chesworth BM, Davis AM et al (2010) Patient satisfaction after total knee arthroplasty: who is satisfied and who is not? Clin Orthop Relat Res 468:57–63

Cheng T, Pan XY, Mao X et al (2012) Little clinical advantage of computer-assisted navigation over conventional instrumentation in primary total knee arthroplasty at early follow-up. Knee 19:237–245

Dossett HG, Swartz GJ, Estrada NA et al (2012) Kinematically versus mechanically aligned total knee arthroplasty. Orthopedics 35:e160–169

Eckhoff DG, Bach JM, Spitzer VM et al (2003) Three-dimensional morphology and kinematics of the distal part of the femur viewed in virtual reality. Part II. J Bone Joint Surg Am 85:97–104

Gothesen O, Espehaug B, Havelin L et al (2011) Short-term outcome of 1,465 computer-navigated primary total knee replacements 2005-2008. Acta Orthop 82:293–300

Hollister AM, Jatana S, Singh AK et al (1993) The axes of rotation of the knee. Clin Orthop Relat Res290:259–268

Howell SM, Kuznik K, Hull ML et al (2008) Results of an initial experience with custom-fit positioning total knee arthroplasty in a series of 48 patients. Orthopedics 31:857–863

Insall JN (1988) Presidential address to The Knee Society. Choices and compromises in total knee arthroplasty. Clin Orthop Relat Res 226:43–48

Jeffery RS, Morris RW, Denham RA (1991) Coronal alignment after total knee replacement. J Bone Joint Surg Br 73:709–714

Lee GC, Lotke PA (2012) Can surgeons predict what makes a good TKA? Intraoperative surgeon impression of TKA quality does not correlate with Knee Society scores. Clin Orthop Relat Res 470:159–165

Magnussen RA, Weppe F, Demey G et al (2011) Residual varus alignment does not compromise results of TKAs in patients with preoperative varus. Clin Orthop Relat Res 469:3443–34450

Parratte S, Pagnano MW, Trousdale RT et al (2010) Effect of postoperative mechanical axis alignment on the fifteen-year survival of modern, cemented total knee replacements. J Bone Joint Surg Am 92:2143–2149

Ritter MA, Faris PM, Keating EM et al (1994) Postoperative alignment of total knee replacement. Its effect on survival. Clin Orthop Relat Res 299:153–156

Spencer BA, Mont MA, McGrath MS et al (2009) Initial experience with custom-fit total knee replacement: intra-operative events and long-leg coronal alignment. Int Orthop 33:1571–1575

Innovations in Navigation of TKA

TKA Navigation Using the Medacta System

Gary D. Botimer

Since its inception over a decade ago, the goal of more accurate prosthesis placement has routinely been met (Bäthis et al. 2004a, 2004b; Bohling et al. 2005; Chauhan et al. 2004a, 2004b; Chin et al. 2005; Krackow et al. 2003; Oberst et al. 2003; Saragaglia et al. 2001; Sparmann et al. 2003; Stulberg et al. 2000, 2002). Although the original prediction of higher longevity with more accurate placement and even distribution of forces has not yet been proven, a meta-analysis of 29 studies of computer-assisted surgery (CAS) vs. standard mechanically instrumented total knee arthroplasty (TKA) showed that errors of 3° occurred in 9% of the former procedures vs. 31.8% of the latter. The controversy over the importance of ±3° mechanical alignment owing to varying midterm reports still does not change the consequences of performing a reconstruction inaccurately nor the ability for CAS to be more accurate (Alden and Pagnano 2008; Berend et al. 2004; Haaker et al. 2005; Mason et al. 2007; Nuno-Siebrecht et al. 2000; Ranawat and Boachie-Adjei 1988; Ritter et al. 2004; Sharkey et al. 2002; Stern and Insall 1992; Teter et al. 1995; Wiese et al. 2004; Wixson 2004). However, this focus may miss the most significant issue remaining in influencing the functional outcome of the new knee. As results have improved, patient expectations have increased. Today's patients, independent of age, expect to live more active lives. This author works in one of the world's »blue zones.« (A *blue zone* is a region of the world where people commonly live active lives past the age of 100 years.) Thus, while the statistics show that the mortality rate after TKA is 3% per year, most of today's patients are not only encouraged but also expect to live physically active lives. This aims the focus toward longevity and stability. While instability remains one of the top three leading causes of early TKA revision (Fehring et al. 2001; Haaker et al. 2005), it also remains one of the leading causes of dissatisfaction in recipients of TKA. After accomplishing the initial goal of fewer mechanical alignment outliers, the real advantage of navigation involves the ability of the system to aid the surgeon in obtaining well-balanced knees throughout the functional range of motion (ROM). We will discuss this further as we describe the surgical technique. During the early 1990s, minimally invasive surgery (MIS) techniques were shown to improve early ROM, reduce blood loss, and decrease hospital stay (Boerger et al. 2005; Haas et al. 2004; Han et al. 2008; Karachalios et al. 2008; Laskin 2007; Pagnano and Meneghini 2006; Schroer et al. 2008) but the complication rate also increased. The major issues have been component malposition, cement removal, and soft tissue injury with malposition being the major occurrence (Dalury and Dennis 2005; Huang et al. 2007) This is exactly where a marriage between navigation and MIS can help significantly.

As with other systems, the CAS instruments are specifically designed to decrease the stress on the soft tissues. In over 5 years of MIS–CAS–TKA, to date we have not had an avulsed patellar tendon but have had a 0.5% incidence of partial or complete medial collateral ligament (MCL) injuries.

The Medacta system is provided cost free to the hospital, but there is a small fee for the disposable reflective balls. Otherwise there is no additional cost. The system is based on the Medacta cutting blocks and as such is tied to their prosthesis. As with most systems, there is an addition of 7–10 min to the overall surgical time once the surgeon is familiar with the system (on average <10 cases). The shorter learning curve is in part related to a strong educational program with visiting surgeons on location and to the way the system is designed. The system has purposely streamlined and simplified the steps as well as the visual presentation of data so as to provide only that information which is needed and can be readily used by the surgeon. The flow and options are also customizable to the surgeon's preference, making the learning curve much shorter. All these subtile issues become more important when we ask the non-CAS and non-MIS surgeon to not only add CAS but also MIS techniques to their skill set.

8.1 System Specifics

The Medacta CAS system is an imageless system using optical balls on the trackers and an infrared camera. There are several features designed to make the system easier to use. The flow is customizable and can be saved in multiple set-ups for each surgeon so that he/she can have the freedom to adjust their technique to fit the patient without having to go through a tedious set-up each time.

The layout of the screens provides a consistent visual feedback with all the necessary information

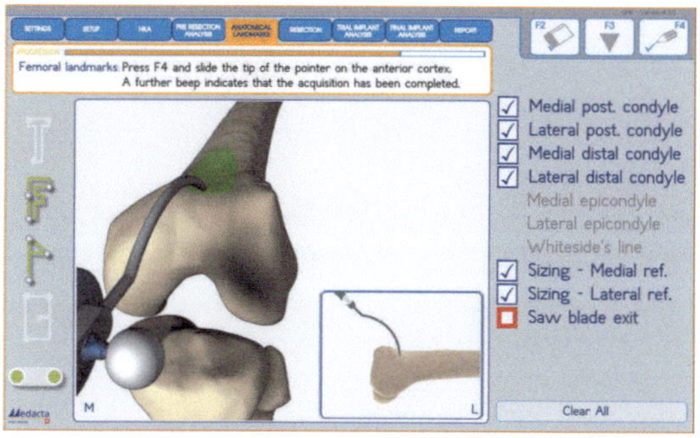

Fig. 8.1 Screenshot of Medacta CAS system showing external rotation of 3° and the estimate of distal resection high at the condyles

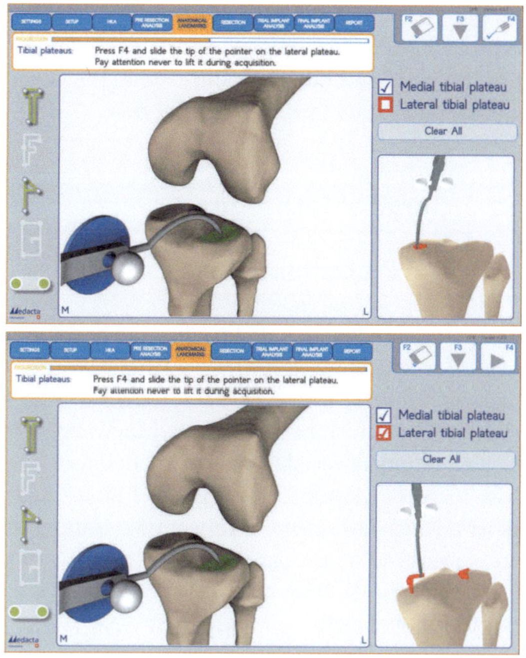

a

b

Fig. 8.2 a,b Double-sided mobile trackers

and intentionally no more (Fig. 8.1). The left-hand side of the screen has a visual of the trackers that are green if seen by the camera. If the surgeon is in the process of acquiring data and the tracker is not recognized by the camera, the tracker image is no longer green and an audible signal alerts the surgeon to the problem. Since femoral and tibial tracker stability is essential for accurate outcomes with CAS systems, the femoral and tibial trackers can be checked at any time on any screen simply by touching the mobile tracker back to the initial reference point established at the beginning of data collection. A number appears next to the tracker image on the left-hand side of the screen to show if, and how much, the tracker has moved.

The mobile trackers are double sided making it easier for the surgeon to obtain the data without having to do as much manipulation of the trackers to obtain camera visualization. The graphics are in real time and modified based on the data provided by the surgeon. This feature provides rapid visual feedback so the surgeon can see if he has accidentally entered an erroneous data point (Fig. 8.2). The disparity from what the surgeon is seeing on the patient and on the screen is readily apparent so that re-registration of the data can be done if necessary. All data collection steps are independent (a specific registration can be recollected at any time without affecting the rest of the registrations). This is very useful when anatomical variations become apparent and/or recollection of a particular data point becomes desirable.

The lower right-hand side of the screen shows the current surgical step and the instruments needed so that the surgical team can better assist the surgeon. The center of the screen provides the surgeon with the information needed for the current step (this is discussed in more detail in Sect. 8.2, »Surgical Technique«). ROM and ligament stability grafts are collected before resection, optionally at the time of trial component placement, and at the conclusion of the case. Any additional information can be added to the case report provided at the end of the case digitally for storage or entry into the medial record. One can record as much or as little as the surgeon desires including any or all steps of the case as well as the grafts. This system collects the results of the cuts not just the jig alignment, not only to be as accurate as possible but because the information is used for the calculations in the following surgical steps. This system was specifically designed to be MIS compatible. Most patients can have an MIS navigated knee with an arthrotomy from the superior pole of the medial tibial tubercle to 2 cm above the superior pole of the patella. The navigation trackers require an additional 1–1.5 cm arthrotomy over the same procedure done conventionally. The technique is designed so that the surgeon can convert to conventional intramedullary femoral and extramedullary tibial aligned cutting guides at any time throughout the procedure with the same guides to maintain the same feel and flow.

8.2 Surgical Technique

8.2.1 Pin Placement: Tibia

The mobile trackers are calibrated at the beginning of each case by the surgeon or the surgical team to make sure they have not been damaged since the last surgery. The tibial pins can be placed anywhere that facilitates camera visualization while not interfering with the tibial extramedullary guide. I prefer mid-tibial through two 2-mm stab wounds. If the pins are placed at 45° to the sagittal plane mid-tibia, they work out well. We have not had any fractures with this technique so far.

8.2.2 Incision and Exposure

The incision is linear over the middle one-third of the patella with the medial parapatellar MIS arthrotomy the surgeon prefers. The proximal tibial dissection is usually limited to 1 cm below the articular surface, except for the anterior–medial tibia that extends in a triangle to the top of the tibial tubercle.

8.2.3 Pin Placement: Femur

The femoral tracker holder, or pins, are placed wherever the surgeon prefers, but usually such that they exit the wound anterior medially and allow the patella to be displaced laterally.

8.2.4 Screen Display

Once the femoral and tibial trackers are placed, the screen shows the camera field of vision and the trackers to assist in ideal camera placement (◘ Fig. 8.3). If necessary, the camera position can be changed any time. Next, the reference points for the »F« and »T« trackers are established. These will be used to check the accuracy of the trackers if needed. This is followed by collecting the following: the most prominent aspect of the medial malleoli, the tip of the lateral malleoli, the center of the tibia proximally, and center of the femur distally. The center of the hip is based on two sets of three data points (hip adducted, abducted, and flexed). A stop sign-like symbol on the screen, with numeric values, gives information on the confidence and accuracy of the hip center. This is followed by establishing the sagittal plane based on limb alignment with the knee extended and flexed. Registration of the tibial plateaus, the posterior and distal femoral condyles, and the anterior femoral cortex as well as the optional registration of the femoral epicondyles, femoral width, and Whiteside's line can be made at the surgeon's discretion. This is especially important in soft tissue balancing. Careful attention to the information allows one to achieve a tight well-balanced knee with ROM of 0–125+ in most cases (◘ Fig. 8.4a, b). In addition to understanding the initial graft, this system has incorporated the use of kinematic measurements of the femoral condyles (◘ Fig. 8.5) and the ability to establish the tibial axis of rotation about the femur, which has been shown to not be the same as the epicondylar line (Churchill et al. 1998; Eckhoff et al. 2005, 2007; Hollister et al. 1993; Howell et al. 2010) It has been my experience that with accurate mechanical alignment, soft tissue releases outside of the posterior capsule in fixed flexion contracture have become rare.

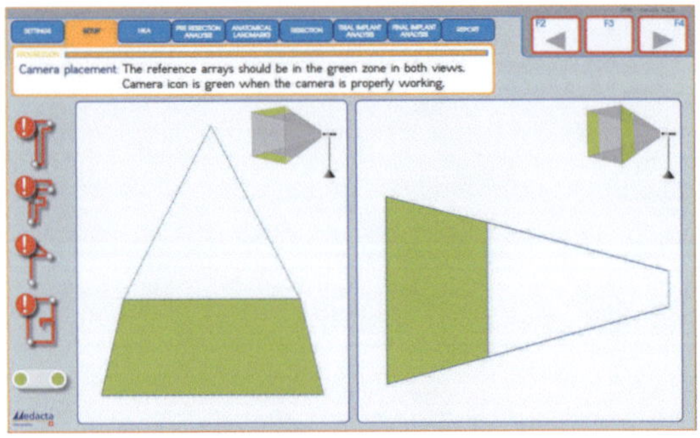

◘ **Fig. 8.3** Screenshot with advice for placement of the infrared camera in the operating theater

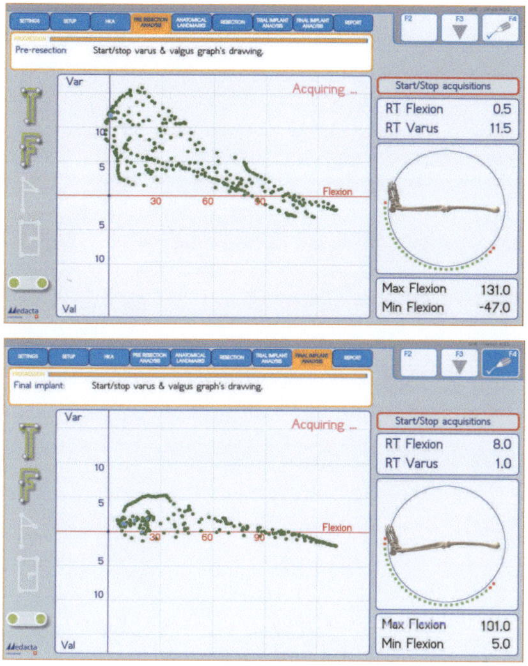

a

b

Fig. 8.4 a,b A tight well-balanced knee with a range of motion of 0–125+ can be achieved in most cases

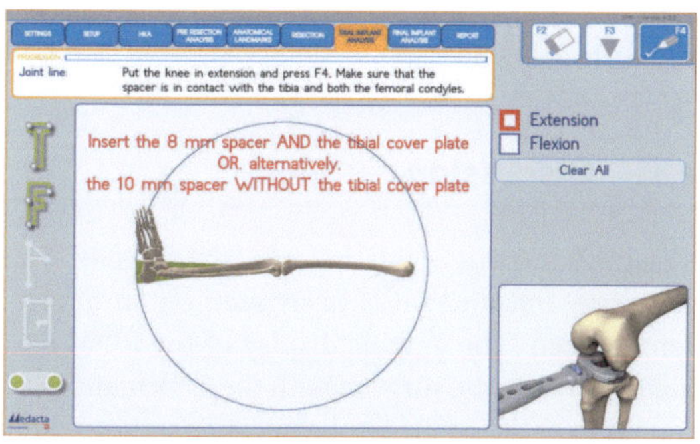

Fig. 8.5 Kinematic measurements of the femoral condyles are incorporated in the system

8.2.5 Placing Cutting Guides

Proximal Tibia

The surgeon can select a distal femoral cut or a proximal tibial cut first. The extramedullary tibial cutting guide is designed to be temporarily pinned with one central pin in the anterior cruciate ligament (ACL) footprint area. The surgeon then navigates the medial-sided cutting guide (or larger cutting guide for a non-MIS approach) into place and pins the cutting block. The initial fixation threaded pin is removed from the ACL footprint and the rest of the extramedullary guide is left in place (Fig. 8.6). This allows the slope and axial alignment to be further adjusted after pinning. It also adds considerably to the stability of the cutting block. The postcut proximal tibial surface is registered.

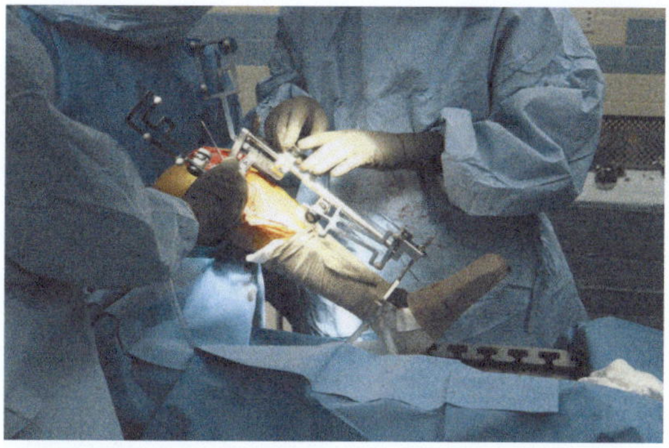

Fig. 8.6 The initial fixation threaded pin is removed from the anterior cruciate ligament footprint with the rest of the extramedullary guide left in place

Distal Femur

The distal femoral micrometric cutting guide is temporarily pinned to the distal condyles. The distal femoral cutting guide is navigated into place using the micrometric guide and pinned (Fig. 8.7). Each of the cutting blocks can be hand positioned and pinned, but the micrometric guides make it much easier and quicker in most surgeons' hands. Once the distal femoral cutting block is pinned, the micrometric guides are removed and the cut is made with or without a saw capture. The femoral cut is registered and used to match the anterior cut length to the component size. This helps prevent long cut run-out in the anterior cortex of the femur past the flange that can lead to bone resorption/notching. At this point, I like to go back and recapture the posterior femoral condyle, because with an MIS technique it is easier to be more accurate at this time. As previously mentioned, any part of the registration can be done independently of the others. The 4-in-1 femoral cutting guide is attached to the distal femoral cutting block with another micrometric guide and the block navigated into the desired

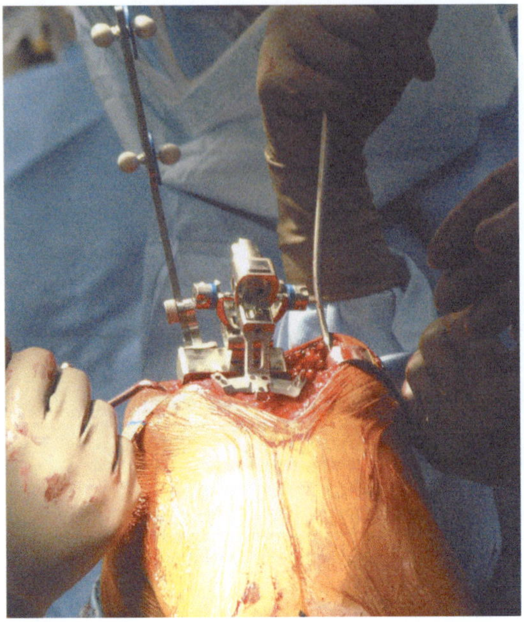

Fig. 8.7 The distal femoral cutting guide is navigated into place using the micrometric guide

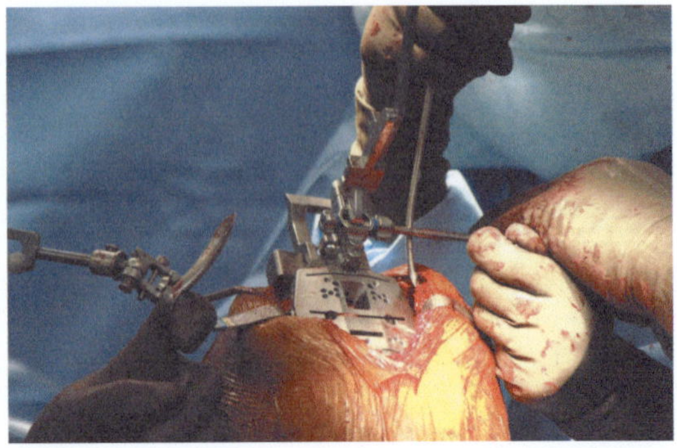

Fig. 8.8 Close-up of navigated 4-in-1 cutting guide

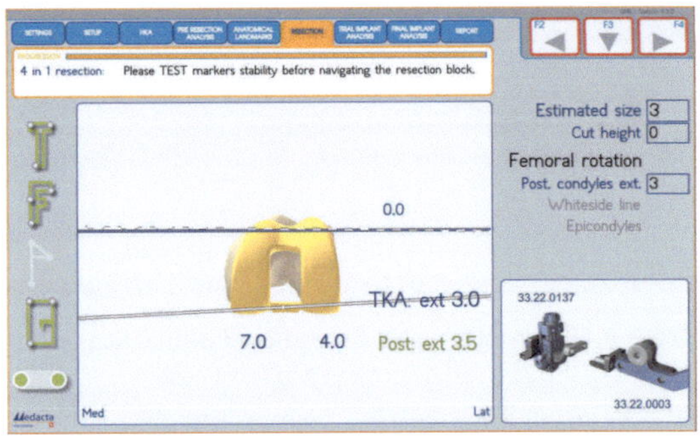

Fig. 8.9 Navigation screen corresponding to the 4-in-1 cutting guide of Figure 8.8

femoral rotation and the anterior cut set at the anterior distal femoral cortex (Fig. 8.8). The block is pinned and the micrometric guide removed or alternately hand positioned, again depending on the surgeon's preference. With the 4-in-1 cutting guide pinned in place and the knee at 90° flexion, the flexion gap can be inspected relative to the rotation of the cutting block to confirm your selection and the distal femoral condylar cuts vs. the purposed posterior cuts. The amount of posterior condyles to be removed is displayed on the screen numerically under the graphic of the posterior condyles. There is also both numeric rotation information as well as a target line to set the rotation to. The target line is set by the surgeon as to his/her preference prior to the case (Fig. 8.9). The tibial and femoral trials are placed in the usual fashion and a graft can be obtained before commitment to the final components. A final graft is then obtained and any additional notes are added. Surgeons can retain as much or as little information as they like. It can be stored in a variety of digital formats.

8.3 Discussion

The specific focus of this system is the surgeon. The necessary information is easily seen on an uncluttered screen. The graphic display of the ROM and laxity provides the surgeon with the information required to make soft tissue balancing decisions with clarity. Surgeons can use measured resection and gap balancing, and they can kinematically establish the tibial axis of rotation about the femur or any combination they desire with the same flow surgically and on graphic displays. The joint line can be monitored pre- and postoperatively for comparison. Registering of the actual cut surfaces and not assuming the cut was the same as the guide all help the surgeon perfect the surgery. Micrometric guides for cutting block positioning alleviate some of the frustrations and improve the fine adjustments. In the end, navigation is a tool to assist the surgeon in obtaining the desired outcome consistently. It is often said that the best system for a surgeon is the one they are most familiar with. The goal of a navigation system should be to accommodate the surgeon and not vice versa. The navigation system should also provide objective information to the surgeon so that they can continually advance the art of total knee replacement. This has been my experience to date with the systems I have used for a decade, including the current system.

References

Alden KJ, Pagnano MW (2008) The consequences of mal-alignment: Are there any? Orthopedics 31:947–948

Bäthis H, Perlick L, Tingart M, Lüring C, Perlick C, Grifka J (2004a) Radiological results of image-based and non-image-based computer-assisted total knee arthroplasty. Int Orthop 28:87–90

Bäthis H, Perlick L, Tingart M, Lüring C, Zurakowski D, Grifka J (2004b) Alignment in total knee arthroplasty: A comparison of computer-assisted surgery with the conventional technique. J Bone Joint Surg Br 86:682–687

Berend ME, Ritter MA, Meding JB, Faris PM, Keating EM, Redelman R, Faris GW, Davis KE (2004) Tibial component failure mechanisms in total knee arthroplasty. Clin Orthop Relat Res 428:26–34

Boerger TO, Aglietti P, Mondanelli N, Sensi L (2005) Mini-subvastus versus medial parapatellar approach in total knee arthroplasty. Clin Orthop Relat Res 440:82–87

Bohling U, Schamberger H, Grittner U, Scholz J (2005) Computerized and technical navigation in total knee arthroplasty. J Orthop Traumatol 5:69

Chauhan SK, Clark GW, Lloyd S, Scott RG, Breidahl W, Sikorski JM (2004a) Computer-assisted total knee replacement. A controlled cadaver study using a multi-parameter quantitative CT assessment of alignment (the Perth CT Protocol). J Bone Joint Surg Br 86:818–823

Chauhan SK, Scott RG, Breidahl W, Beaver RJ (2004b) Computer-assisted knee arthroplasty versus a conventional jig-based technique. A randomised, prospective trial. J Bone Joint Surg Br 86:372–377

Chin PL, Yang KY, Yeo SJ, Lo NN (2005) Randomized control trial comparing radiographic total knee arthroplasty implant placement using computer navigation versus conventional technique. J Arthroplasty 20:618–626

Churchill DL, Incavo SJ, Johnson CC, Beynnon BD (1998) The transepicondylar axis approximates the optimal flexion axis of the knee. Clin Orthop Relat Res 356:111–118

Dalury DF, Dennis DA (2005) Mini-incision total knee arthroplasty can increase risk of component malalignment. Clin Orthop Relat Res 440:77–81

Eckhoff DG, Bach JM, Spitzer VM, Reinig KD, Bagur MM, Baldini TH, Flannery NM (2005) Three-dimensional mechanics, kinematics, and morphology of the knee viewed in virtual reality. J Bone Joint Surg Am 87:71–80

Eckhoff D, Hogan C, DiMatteo L, Robinson M, Bach J (2007) Difference between the epicondylar and cylindrical axis of the knee. Clin Orthop Relat Res 461:238–244

Fehring TK, Odum S, Griffin WL, Mason JB, Nadaud M (2001) Early failures in total knee arthroplasty. Clin Orthop Relat Res 392:315–318

Haaker RG, Stockheim M, Kamp M, Prof G, Breitenfelder J, Ottersbach A (2005) Computer navigation increases precision in component placement in TKA. Clin Orthop 433:152–159

Haas SB, Cook S, Beksac B (2004) Minimally invasive total knee replacement through a mini midvastus approach: A comparative study. Clin Orthop Relat Res 428:68–73

Han I, Seong SC, Lee S, Yoo JH, Lee MC (2008) Simultaneous bilateral MIS-TKA results in faster functional recovery. Clin Orthop Relat Res 466:1449–1453

Hollister AM, Jatana S, Singh AK, Sullivan WW, Lupichuk AG (1993) The axes of rotation of the knee. Clin Orthop Relat Res 290:259–268

Howell SM, Howell SJ, Hull ML (2010) Assessment of the radii of the medial and lateral femoral condyles in varus and valgus knees with osteoarthritis. J Bone Joint Surg Am 92:98–104

Huang HT, Su JY, Chang JK, Chen CH, Wang GJ (2007) The early clinical outcome of minimally invasive quadriceps-sparing total knee arthroplasty: Report of a 2-year follow-up. J Arthroplasty 22:1007–1012

Karachalios T, Giotikas D, Roidis N, Poultsides L, Bargiotas K, Malizos KN (2008) Total knee replacement performed with either a mini-midvastus or a standard approach: A prospective randomised clinical and radiological trial. J Bone Joint Surg Br 90:584–591

Krackow KA, Phillips MJ, Bayers-Thering M, Serpe L, Mihalko WM (2003) Computer-assisted total knee arthroplasty: navigation in TKA. Orthopedics 26:1017–1023

Laskin RS (2007) Surgical exposure for total knee arthroplasty: for everything there is a season. J Arthroplasty 22S:12–14

Mason JB, Fehring TK, Estok R, Banel D, Fahrbach K (2007) Meta-analysis of alignment outcomes in computer-assisted total knee arthroplasty surgery. J Arthroplasty 22:1097–1106

Mulhall KJ, Ghomrawi HM, Scully S, Callaghan JJ, Saleh KJ (2006) Current etiologies and modes of failure in total knee arthroplasty revision. Clin Orthop Relat Res 446:45–50

Nuno-Siebrecht N, Tanzer M, Bobyn JD (2000) Potential errors in axial alignment using intramedullary instrumentation for total knee arthroplasty. J Arthroplasty 15:228–230

Oberst M, Bertsch C, Würstlin S, Holz U (2003) CT analysis of leg alignment after conventional vs. navigated knee prosthesis implantation: Initial results of a controlled, prospective and randomized study. Unfallchirurg 106:941–948

Pagnano MW, Meneghini RM (2006) Minimally invasive total knee arthroplasty with an optimized subvastus approach. J Arthroplasty 21S:22–26

Ranawat CS, Boachie-Adjei O (1988) Survivorship analysis and results of total condylar knee arthroplasty. Clin Orthop 226:6–13

Ritter MA, Faris PM, Keating EM, Meding JB (1994) Postoperative alignment of total knee replacement. Its effect on survival. Clin Orthop 299:153–156

Saragaglia D, Picard F, Chaussard C, Montbarbon E, Leitner F, Cinquin P (2001) Computer-assisted knee arthroplasty: Comparison with a conventional procedure. Results of 50 cases in a prospective, randomized study. Rev Chir Orthop Reparatrice Appar Mot 87:18–28

Schroer WC, Diesfeld PJ, Reedy ME, LeMarr AR (2008) Mini-subvastus approach for total knee arthroplasty. J Arthroplasty 23:19–25

Sharkey PF, Hozack WJ, Rothman RH, Shastri S, Jacoby SM (2002) Insall Award Paper: Why are total knee arthroplasties failing today? Clin Orthop 404:7–13

Sparmann M, Wolke B, Czupalla H, Banzer D, Zink A (2003) Positioning of total knee arthroplasty with and without navigation support. A prospective, randomized study. J Bone Joint Surg Br 85:830–835

Stern SH, Insall JN (1992) Posterior stabilized prosthesis: Results after follow-up of 9–12 years. J Bone Joint Surg Am 74:980–986

Stulberg DS, Picard F, Saragaglia D (2000) Computer-assisted total knee replacement arthroplasty. Oper Tech Orthop 10:25

Stulberg SD, Loan PB, Sarin V (2002) Computer-assisted navigation in total knee replacement: results of an initial experience in thirty-five patients. J Bone Joint Surg Am 84S:90–98

Teter KE, Bergman D, Colwell CW (1995) Accuracy of intramedullary versus extramedullary tibial alignment cutting systems in total knee arthroplasty. Clin Orthop 321:106–110

Wiese M, Rosenthal A, Bernsmann K (2004) Clinical experience using the SurgiGATE system. In: Stiehl JB, Konermann WH, Haaker RG (eds) Navigation and robotics in total joint and spine surgery. Springer, Berlin Heidelberg New York Tokyo, pp. 400–404

Wixson RL (2004) Extra-medullary computer assisted total knee replacement: towards lesser invasive surgery. In: Stiehl JB, Konermann WH, Haaker RG (eds) Navigation and robotics in total joint and spine surgery. Springer, Berlin Heidelberg New York Tokyo, pp. 311–318

Total Knee Revision Supported by the OrthoPilot® Navigation System

Ulrich Clemens

Total knee arthroplasty (TKA) has become a success story. Nevertheless, today there are a growing number of arthroplasties that have to be revised. The revision of knee arthroplasty is a challenging procedure. During the last 20 years, there have been significant improvements in the development of implants, instruments, and strategies for revision. Additionally, navigation has assumed a growing role in primary TKA. It has been shown that navigation results in a superior alignment to that of manual implantation (Bäthis et al. 2004; Jenny and Boeri 2001). Achieving perfect alignment is one of the major challenges in revision arthroplasty, and consequently B. Braun Aesculap launched a total knee revision (TKR) version of their navigation system OrthoPilot® in October 2008.

9.1 Method

The OrthoPilot® navigation system forces the surgeon to plan. As should be done in a manual revision, the surgeon has to answer the following questions:

Why did the first surgery fail?

- Was the implant bad?
- Has the first implant done its job?
- Was there infection?
- Was the cementless implant a failure?
- Was there failure in cementing?
- Did polyethylene wear occur?
- Was there allergy?
- Malpositioning of the components:
  - Where is the joint line?
  - Where is the height of the patella?
  - Rotation of the femoral component?
  - Rotation of the tibial component?
  - Correct size of the components?

The surgeon has to look for additional sources of information

- Surgical report of the first surgery
- X-rays before the first surgery
- X-ray of the opposite knee
- Spiral computed tomography (CT) scan to check or quantify the malrotation

With all the information on hand, the surgeon has to decide on the aims

- Which size is planned for the femoral and tibial component?
- Where should the joint line be?
- Is the rotational alignment of the femoral and tibial component correct, or should it be changed? If so, by how much?
- Is there a need for stem extensions? Can they be cementless or cemented? Are there problems related to curved bones, lying implants, or screws?
- Is there a need for any augments or bone graft?

9.2 Workflow of OrthoPilot® TKR 1.0

A normal wide opening of the joint is made. Synovectomy follows, if necessary. The rigid bodies are mounted onto the femur and the tibia. For the femoral side, a special C-clamp has been developed so there is no conflict with the planned intramedullary stem. On the tibial side, the author prefers a bicortical fixation below the planned tibial stem. A monocortical fixation is also offered by the manufacturer.

After starting the software, the system asks for the patient's name, the operated side, and the planned implant. The next question concerns the planned joint line. The system asks for a reference point and the planned distance to the reference point. For example: If the surgeon wants 5 mm distalization of the femoral component, he has to fill in »5 mm distal to the femoral reference.« Later in the workflow, the surgeon has to palpate the point that is to be distalized, the most distal part of the femoral component (Fig. 9.1).

The next step is the kinematic acquisition of the hip, ankle, and knee joint. Additionally, the surgeon has to palpate a few points very carefully and keep in mind what the task of the palpated point is in the workflow. The midpoint of the current tibial implant has to be palpated. The palpated point is the top of the mechanical axis of the tibia. It should not be a problem to find the midpoint of the tray. This point is linked to the calculated center of the ankle, and the tibial resection block is orientated perpendicular to this line. After palpation of the tibial midpoint, the tibial implant can be removed. Then, the

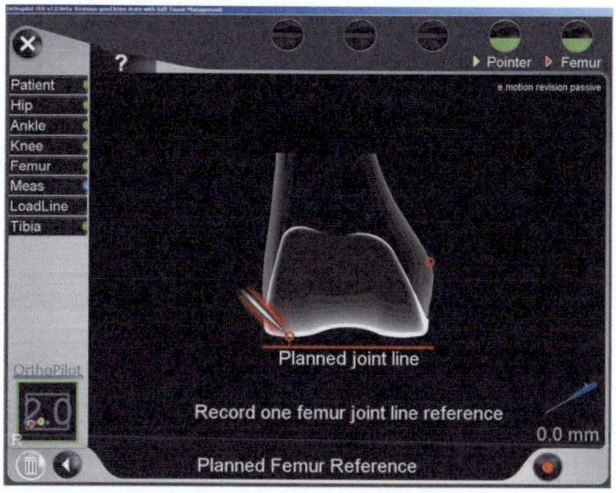

Fig. 9.1 The screen asks the surgeon to palpate the reference point on the femur from which he has calculated his future joint line

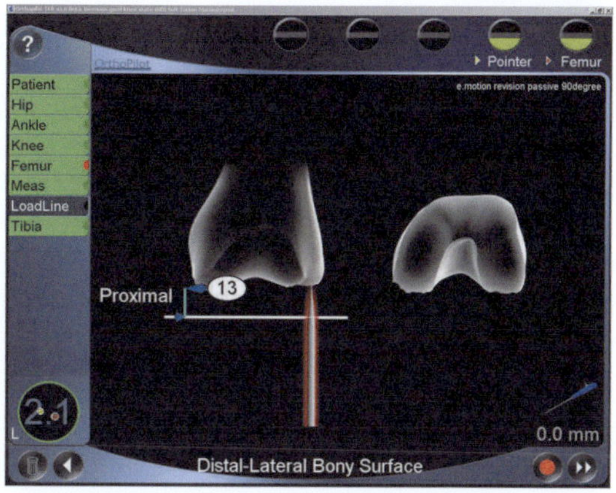

Fig. 9.2 One of four screens for palpating the defect situation on the femoral side. The *number 13* on the screen indicates 13 mm and is the distance from the palpated point to the planned distal joint line. Since 13 mm cannot be filled with the femoral component alone, augments have to be considered

tibial defects on the medial and lateral side are palpated and the resection screen shows the surgeon the resection height on the tibia in relation to these two palpated points. If the intended cut is above the palpated point, the distance is indicated in yellow. This should be kept in mind if one is dealing with contained or uncontained defects. If the cutting block is perfectly positioned, the surgeon makes the cut perpendicular to the mechanical tibial axis. From this perfectly orientated bottom of the flexion and extension gap, the stem extension can be prepared. The author prefers short cemented stems in order to keep the perfect position of the tibial and femoral component. Additional cemented stems have been shown to have superior results in revision (Fehring et al. 2003). Cementless stems sometimes lead to a malalignment of the component because they are guided by the intramedullary canal (Laskin 2003).

Under the guidance of the OrthoPilot® system, the posterior condylar line of the current femoral component is now palpated. From the preoperative CT scan, the surgeon knows that, for example, an additional 7° of external rotation is needed. With the orienting block, the surgeon enters this value as a default in the system. The surgeon then palpates the anterior cortex of the femur laterally at the proximal end of the femoral component. This point will be the rotating axis of the femoral component parallel to the mechanical axis. Additionally, the dorsal palpated points provide the final information on the size of the component. This can be compared with the planned size, coming from a template on the x-ray of the knee before the first operation or from an x-ray of the opposite side. The surgeon's idea of the size becomes more solid.

The femoral component is now removed and the defect situation of the medial and lateral femur is palpated. The surgeon palpates two points distally and two points dorsally. As the surface of the palpated area is not flat, it is up to the surgeon to palpate on a mountain or in a valley of the surface. However, the point of palpation should be kept in mind in order to reach a perfect position for the cutting block. By palpating distally, the distance of this point from the intended joint line is indicated (Fig. 9.2). If at this point 12 mm, for example, is shown on the screen, the surgeon knows that a normal implant is not thick enough. One then has to calculate with augmentations. For example, if you have an implant with a thickness of 9 mm, you will make an additional cut of 1 mm and you will need a 4-mm block. The nurse can start preparing the instruments and the trial implants in this early stage.

Now the extension gap is measured. During the measurement, the resulting varus/valgus angulation is indicated. If the value is 4 or lower, the

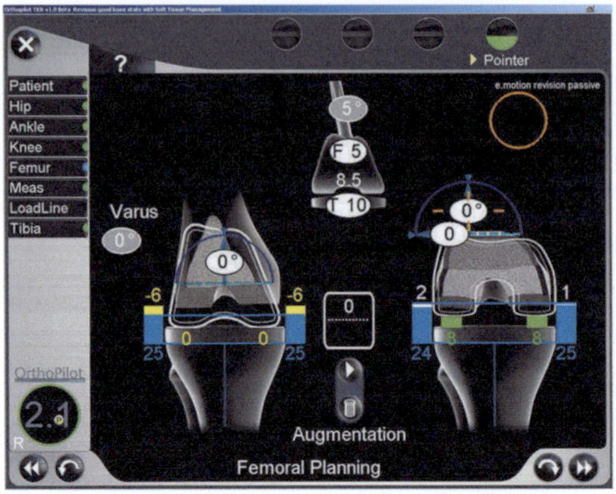

▪ **Fig. 9.3** The planning screen. On the *left side* the situation in extension is simulated, on the *right side* the situation in flexion. In the *middle* (*top part*), the component sizes are shown (in this case a femur of size 5 with a distal thickness of 8.5 mm and a tibial component with a total thickness of 10 mm). Below, the component inside the *square* is the distance from the planned distal joint line. The screen is shown after measuring the extension gap (*left side*) and flexion gap (*right side*). The values are indicated in *blue numbers* and *columns*. On *top* of the *blue columns*, the amount of bone that has to be resected is indicated in *white* (*right side*) or the missing bone is indicated in *yellow* (*left side*) as a trigger for necessary augments

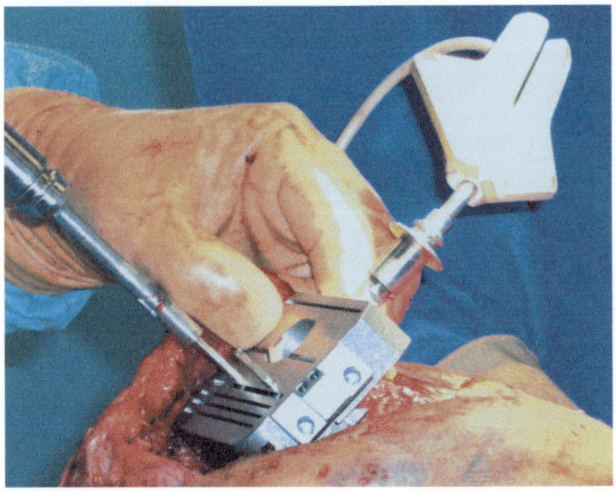

▪ **Fig. 9.4** The navigated 4-in-1 block with distal augments is positioned to the femoral distal resection. Under control of navigation, the perfect anteroposterior position and rotation is found and the position is fixed with pins

surgeon can proceed. If the value is higher, the surgeon should consider a release to balance the knee up to a value of 4 or less. Over-release has to be avoided. The gaps are stored in the system and the flexion gap is measured. Once stored in the system, the OrthoPilot® changes to the planning screen (▪ Fig. 9.3).

The planning screen is developed from the primary TKA navigation. The planned joint line is integrated in the middle of the screen. OrthoPilot® as a default starts with no distance to the planned joint line, and a value of 0. If the relevant parameters are changed, the new distance to the planned joint line is shown. A second new feature is the indication of the cutting height. If there is no bone behind the cutting block, the distance to the bone is indicated in yellow. This means there is a need for a metal step, a bone graft, or filling with cement. In a hidden screen the surgeon can plan the steps distally and dorsally on the medial and lateral side and the nurse can prepare the trial implants.

On the planning screen (▪ Fig. 9.3) the surgeon plans all the femoral cuts, the definite femoral size, the femoral rotation, the femoral and tibial augments, and the height of the tibial onlay. After the definite plan, the next step is distal femoral resection. The navigated resection block is positioned perpendicular to the mechanical axis of the femur, and the surgeon has the option of performing the resection medially and laterally and preparing the distal steps with respect to the planned joint line. The distal resection is controlled by the navigated 4-in-1 resection block with the planned augments in their definite position (▪ Fig. 9.4). If the resected plan is perfect, the navigated resection block is rotated to the planned position and finally the anteroposterior position is adjusted. In this position the block will be carefully fixed and the four cuts can be made. Meanwhile, the trial implants are prepared by the nurse and the final check can be made; the mechanical axis is controlled by the navigation as is the range of motion. If everything is fine, preparation of the stem can start.

The navigation system offers a second way forward, coming from perfectly aligned stems. Most of the manual revision systems work with an alignment strategy resulting from intramedullary guiding. A well-fitting intramedullary stem is prepared and the cutting block is mounted onto this stable stem, which is positioned in the tibia or femur. The OrthoPilot® TKR 1.0 supports this procedure with

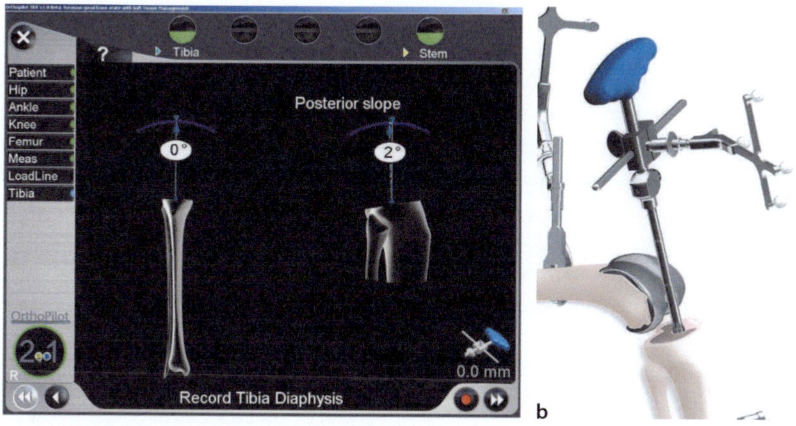

a b

Fig. 9.5a,b A rigid body is mounted on the reamer. While reaming, the surgeon has control over varus/valgus angulation and slope. (By courtesy of B. Braun, Aesculap)

navigated reaming of the stem (Fig. 9.5). A rigid body is mounted on the reamer and the surgeon is able to control varus/valgus alignment and the slope while reaming. As soon as the reamer has found the final stable position, the instrumentation process continues in the same way as in the manual technique. However, the surgeon has the additional possibility to control the cuts with the help of navigation.

9.3 Experience

To date, the author's experience with this system includes more than 100 navigated revisions. It was very helpful to work with the checklist. After clinical examination and after checking the current x-rays (including a long-leg x-ray), the questions were answered carefully. Restoring the joint line is one of the main issues in TKR. If the joint line is raised, the clinical rating scores go down. But unfortunately in TKR there is a general tendency to raise the joint line (Partington et al. 1999). For each millimeter that the joint line is raised to its original position, the patellofemoral contact forces increase by 3% (Singerman et al. 1994). Proximalization of the joint line shows a higher rate of instability of the joint (Laskin 2002). Hofmann and coworkers found better flexion, extension, stability, and lower pain scores if the joint line was restored ±4 mm to the natural height compared to those with a distance of more than 4 mm (Hofmann et al. 2006). Where to go with the joint line in revision cases is still an open question. Laskin suggests 25 mm below the medial epicondyle for any revision (Laskin 2002). Hofmann compares the actual joint line with the preoperative x-ray of the same side or the x-ray of the contralateral side, using the medial adductor tubercle as reference point. His mean value for the distance from the medial epicondylar flare to the joint line was 45 mm, with a range from 22 to 63 mm (Hofmann et al. 2006).

Mountney and colleagues in two sophisticated studies found a constant relationship between the transepicondylar axis length (TEAL) and the distance from the medial sulcus to the joint line (MC): TEAL/MC=k=3.4 (Mountney et al. 2007). Mountney requested that this algorithm should be integrated in the navigation software. The algorithm is not included in the TKR 1.0 software, and therefore the author prefers to compare the lateral x-rays with those before the first operation or with those of the contralateral knee. The height of the cartilage was respected. In this way, the necessary change of the joint line height was defined and included in the intro screen. From then on, the guidance of the system was perfect and led to the expected results for the joint line.

A second joint line to be respected is the posterior joint line. Hofmann reports on the restoration of the correct anteroposterior size, which means the same. A smaller component leads to an unstable flexion gap and must be changed. Comparing the original lateral views with the template of the revision system gives a concrete idea of the best size for the femoral component and shows that dorsal augmentation is necessary (Hofmann et al. 2006). Knowing the right size, this value can be introduced in the planning screen and the results for the gaps are then shown by the system.

Rotation of the femoral component is no longer a challenge. Implantation of the component parallel to the transepicondylar axis was regarded as correct. A CT scan with the primary femoral implant was performed, the malpositioning was defined, and the value was introduced into the navigation system. Grafinger and colleagues showed that by using this method in primary TKA, the accuracy of the rotation could be improved very effectively (Grafinger et al. 2008). Michaut and coworkers claimed that the preoperative CT-based method is favorable for a perfect rotational alignment of the femoral component compared to the navigation methods based on intraoperatively palpated epicondyles or Whiteside's line (Michaut et al. 2008). Takai and colleagues described a simple roentgenographic technique in 80° of knee flexion, which shows the transepicondylar axis and the posterior condylar line (Takai et al. 2003). In addition to the planned rotation of the femoral component, the planning screen shows the balance of the resulting flexion gap. The navigation system gives some information including Whiteside's line, and surgeons finally have to decide according to their clinical judgement if there is a conflict.

TKR navigation cannot achieve the same precise values as those achieved in primary TKA with respect to the often weak bone, and it remains a challenge to fixate the rigid bodies and of course the resecting blocks.

9.4 Conclusion

The challenging procedure of TKR is very effectively supported by the OrthoPilot® TKR 1.0 navigation system. With the workflow based on perfect cuts and well-balanced gaps, the author was able to reduce surgery time. Additionally, it was observed, as Hungerford stated in 1993, that with a perfect restoration of the joint line and alignment, the amount of intrinsic constraints can be reduced (Hungerford 1993). Using navigation, the balance of flexion to extension gaps becomes easier and the workflow is more organized than with the manual technique. Revision of TKA remains a challenge and is reserved for surgeons who are experienced in navigation and in the revision of TKA.

References

Bäthis HL, Perlick M, Tingart et al (2004) Alignment in total knee arthroplasty. J Bone Joint Surg Br 86:682–687

Fehring TK, Odum S, Olekson C et al (2003) Stem fixation in revision total knee arthroplasty: a comparative analysis. Clin Orthop Relat Res 416:217–224

Grafinger RW, Datz L, Hitzl W, Dorn U (2008) CT scans increase rotational accuracy in total knee arthroplasty. Z Orthop Unfall 146:782–787

Hofmann A, Kurtin SM, Lyons S et al (2006) Clinical and radiographic analysis of accurate restoration of the joint line in total knee revision arthroplasty. J Arthroplasty 21:1154–1162

Hungerford DS (1993) Revision total knee replacement. Tech Orthop 7:80–85

Jenny JY, Boeri C (2001) Navigated implantation of total knee endoprostheses: a comparative study with conventional instrumentation. Z Orthop Ihre Grenzgeb 139:117–119

Laskin RS (2002) Joint line position restoration during revision total knee replacement. Clin Orthop Relat Res 404:169:–171

Laskin RS (2003) Instrumentation pitfalls: you just can't go to autopilot! J Arthroplasty 18:18–22

Michaut M, Beaufils P, Galaud B et al (2008) Rotational alignment of femoral component with computed assisted surgery (CAS) during total knee arthroplasty. REV Chir Orthop Reparatrice Appar Mot 94:580–584

Mountney J, Karamfiles R, Breidahl W et al (2007) The position of the joint line in relation to the tran-epicondylar axis of the knee. J Arthroplasty 22:1201–1207

Partington PF, Sawhney J, Rorabeck CH et al (1999) Joint line restoration after revision total knee arthroplasty. Clin Orthop Relat Res 367:165–171

Singerman R, Davy DT, Goldberg VM (1994) Effects of patella alta and patella infera on patellofemoral contact forces. J Biomech 27:1059–1065

Takai S, Yoshino N, Isshiki T et al (2003) Kneeling view: a new roentgenographic technique to assess rotational deformity and alignment of the distal femur. J Arthroplasty 18:478–483

Disclosure: The author was involved in the development of the revision software. Additionally he is engaged as an instructor during revision and navigation courses organized by B. Braun, Aesculap.

Brainlab Dash®: iPod®-Based Navigation System in Total Knee and Hip Replacements

Holger Bäthis

Computer-assisted techniques in total joint replacement procedures have been used for more than 10 years, with numerous studies demonstrating superior results regarding implant position and correction of leg deformities compared to conventional techniques. This has been shown both in randomized trials and in large-scale retrospective cohort analyses. Nevertheless, the technique has not become the standard of care in most hospitals around the world. There are several reasons why the navigation technique is still not used regularly despite its valuable advantages. The main obstacles in implementing the technique are undoubtedly the additional costs for the patient, the surgeon, the hospital, or – in view of medical reimbursement systems – even the community. The costs can be divided into direct costs for investment and costs per case or indirect costs such as the additional time required for the surgical procedure. Moreover, the computer-assisted technique is still perceived as a demanding procedure; surgeons require training and need to complete their own learning curve before becoming familiar with the technique compared to the conventional technique that they are already trained in. Based on these conditions, Brainlab AG started a development project in 2007 to tackle some of these obstacles so as to increase general acceptance of the navigation technique in joint replacement surgeries. The main aspects of the development agenda were to create simplified user-friendly software algorithms, intuitive handling, a system with lower investment costs, and an optimized time frame for setting up the system as well as for the surgery itself. Our hospital department joined a development cooperation and we were involved in multiple design reviews, cadaver workshops, and a clinical prototype study on total hip and knee replacement, until the final release of the system.

10.1 Technical Aspects

10.1.1 Dash® Hardware Components

Similar to all modern surgical navigation systems that are used for joint replacement procedures, the Dash® system is an image-free navigation system. All joint information is digitized during the surgery. No specialized preoperative diagnostics are necessary.

In order to create more intuitive workflows, the concept of a handheld navigation device was developed. Moreover, the idea was tested and approved to implement the Apple iPod touch®[1] as a consumer market electronic device into the hardware concept of a medical device, using its widely accepted user interface technology coming from the revolutionary Apple iPhone®.

Central to the hardware concept is a sterile draped iPod touch® with a 3.5-inch touchscreen interface and retina display that is included into a handheld cradle. The iPod® works remotely with a separate computer platform that is included in the infrared camera stand using a secured wireless-LAN network connection. Except for the power supply of the camera system, no further cable connections are necessary, especially no cables within the surgical field.

The system is designed »implant-independently« to be used with any total hip system and various types of knee systems available.

The small number of additional instruments from the Dash® can be attached to the handheld cradle that is equipped with three reflecting marker spheres that are tracked by the infrared camera (◘ Fig. 10.1a,b). These are used for the initial digitalization of the patient's anatomy in the total knee replacement (TKR) cases. For the Dash® hip, only the pointer is necessary.

During the navigation-assisted bone resection and verification, the cradle is attached to the universal resection guides provided by the individual TKR instrumentation set.

All instruments are reusable at minimal costs.

The system is portable with a small base both for easy set up in the operating room (OR) and also for use in different ORs or hospitals in just one transportation case for easy transport (◘ Fig. 10.2).

10.1.2 Concept of Sterile iPod® Implementation

At the beginning of the surgery, the iPod® is covered in a single-use sterile drape, comparable with an ar-

1 iPod®, iPod touch®, and iPhone® are registered trademarks of Apple Inc.

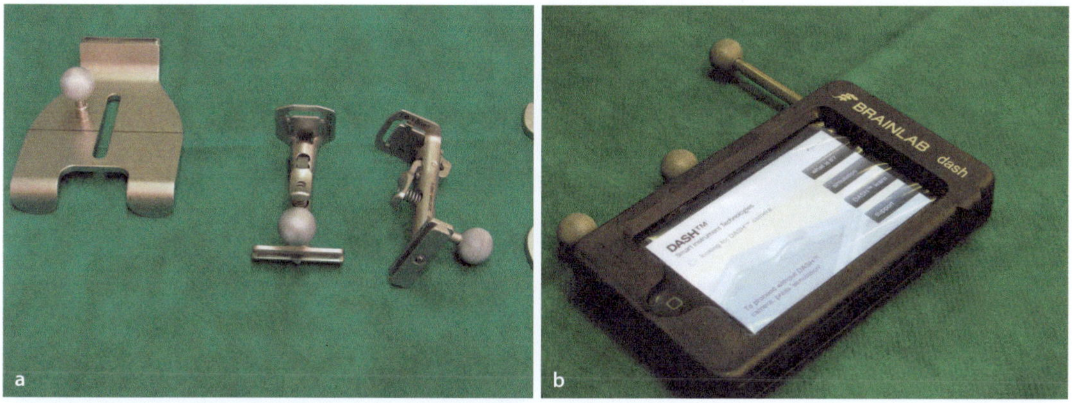

Fig. 10.1 **a** Cradle with draped iPod touch®. **b** Dash® instruments

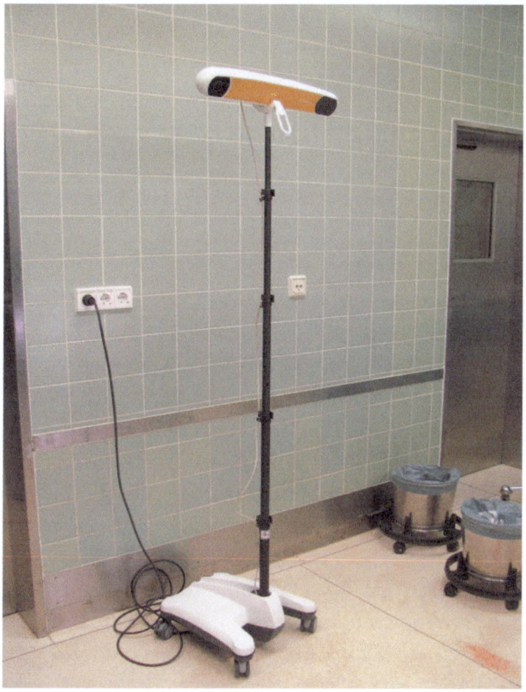

Fig. 10.2 Camera system

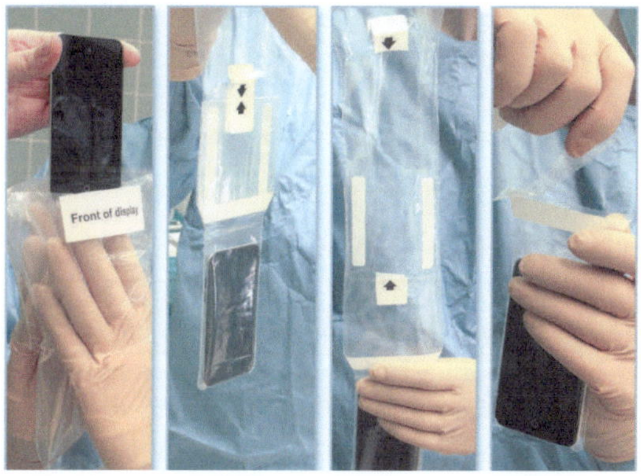

Fig. 10.3 Certified sterile draping of the Apple iPod®

throscopic camera drape. A certified commercial draping was developed, where the device is put into a plastic tube. The special design includes a tube at the end of a clear bag that can be sealed without the risk of contamination (Fig. 10.3). The draped iPod® is placed in the cradle afterwards. With the sterile draping there is only a slight change in the visibility of the display as well as in the touchscreen response.

10.1.3 Dash® Software Workflows

To increase acceptance of the navigation technique, the software workflows were also optimized so as to create more efficient workflows for the surgeon. Some functions that are already available with modern navigation systems, such as bone morphing or ligament balance analysis, were removed in order to focus on the main and proven aspects of the navigation technique.

For both hip and knee applications, simplified algorithms for landmark digitalization have been developed with a significant reduction in the start-up interval. Each navigation step is introduced by a short demonstration clip, which can be skipped if the procedure is clear.

The software app for the iPod® can be downloaded and updated from the Apple iTunes® store

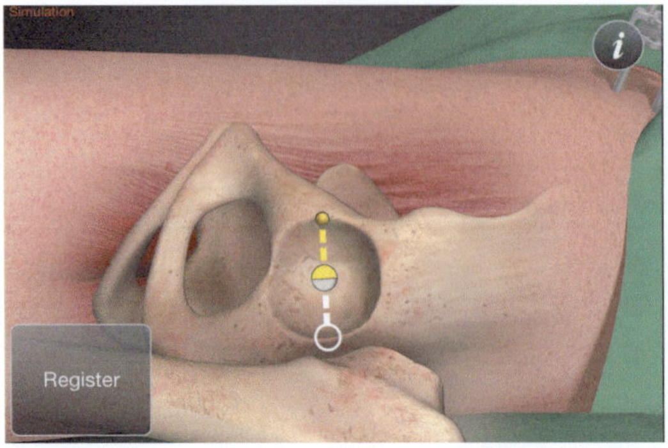

Fig. 10.4 Screenshots of the Landmark hip. (By courtesy of Brainlab AG)

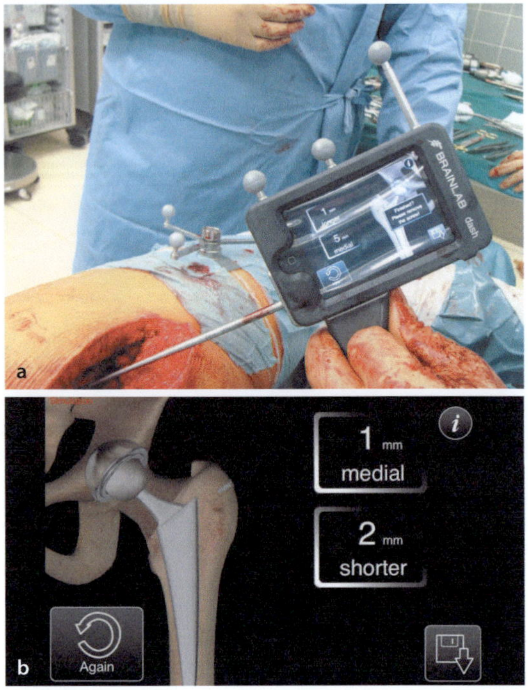

Fig. 10.5 **a** Intraoperative measurement. **b** Screenshot for hip result. (By courtesy of Brainlab AG)

for free. If no camera system is present, the software runs in a simulation modus for preoperative training purposes. In addition, a teaching application (Dash® learn) with training videos is available.

10.1.4 Dash® Hip Application

The Dash® hip application is an intraoperative control system for leg length and femoral offset during total hip replacement (THR). The software can be used with any hip implant system both for primary and revision cases without additional specialized hardware. Surgeries can be performed with the patient in supine and lateral position using any kind of surgical approach without limitation.

In the beginning, a reference array is fixed to the iliac crest using two small Steinmann pins. On the femur no bony fixation of a reference array is necessary, only a short 3.5-mm screw is fixed to the greater trochanter to have a clearly defined reference point for the intraoperative measurements. One additional reference array is placed on top of the distal thigh using an adhesive drape. This array is not used for measurement calculations but to place the leg in similar positions when repeating the leg length measurements.

Only three landmarks have to be digitized to define the preoperative hip geometry. These are the screw head on the greater trochanter (before femoral head luxation/resection) and the anterior and posterior acetabular rim to define the region of the acetabular center (Fig. 10.4).

At this stage the hip replacement is performed as usual until the trial implants are in place. Again the leg is placed in a similar position using the iPod® and the screw head is then digitized again with the iPod Pointer® (Fig. 10.5a).

Instantly the surgeon gets the results of hip geometry with the difference in leg length and offset compared to the pre-operative situation. By changing different head / neck combinations the optimal solution for the patients can be defined and finished with the final implants. With last saved values of leg length and offset a patient report is prepared and stored to the iPod® that can be printed immediately after connecting the iPod® to any computer (Fig. 10.5b).

10.1.5 Dash® Knee Application

For TKR, two different procedures are available. In addition to the standard workflow, a so-called pinless workflow is available, where no additional reference arrays are necessary on the femur and tibia.

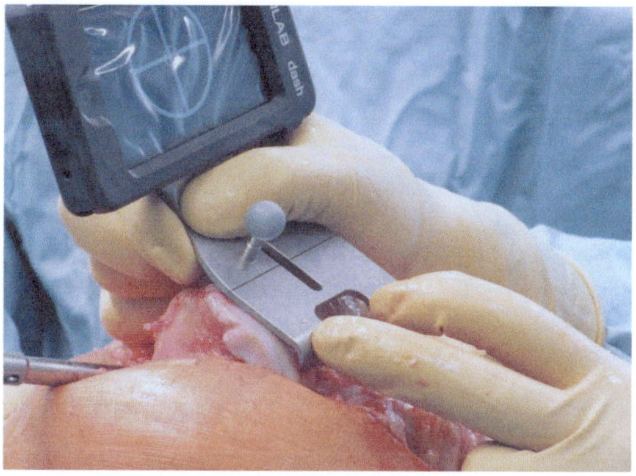

■ **Fig. 10.6** Navigation-guided registration of the distal femur

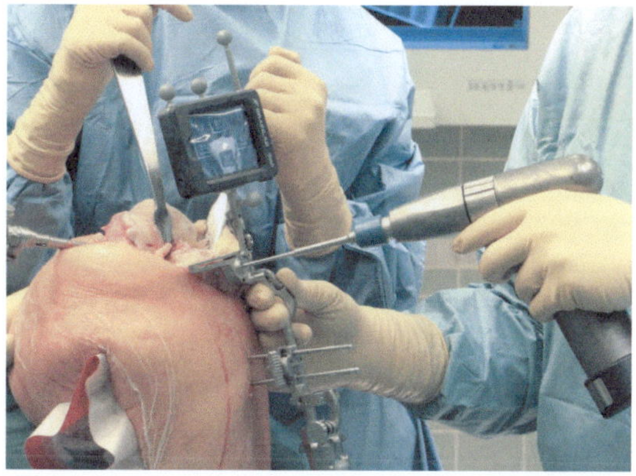

■ **Fig. 10.7** Navigation-based adjustment of proximal tibia resection block

The pinless workflow is available with the Dash® 1.1 software update from October 2012.

10.1.6 Standard Workflow for TKR

The principles of the standard workflow are comparable to the established navigation technique in TKR. After a skin and capsular incision is made, a reference array has to be attached to the distal femur and the tibia. Afterwards, digitalization of a very limited number of anatomic landmarks is necessary. For example, the digitalization of all distal femur landmarks is done within one step using a software-controlled paddle, which is placed on top of the distal femoral condyle (■ Fig. 10.6). This optimized registration process only takes about 2 min of additional OR time. Now the software can be used according to the surgeon's preference, either femur or tibia first. The surgeon is able to perform distal femur or proximal tibial resection at any time and is also able to return to the other resection as needed (■ Fig. 10.7, ■ Fig. 10.8).

For the resection, the iPod® cradle is attached to the cutting block and positioned using the iPod® screen. The surgeon gets instant and comprehensive information on the resection level on the medial and lateral compartment, the flexion/extension position (e.g., slope), and the varus/valgus alignment displayed in clear letters that are visible directly in the surgeon's working direction and field of interest.

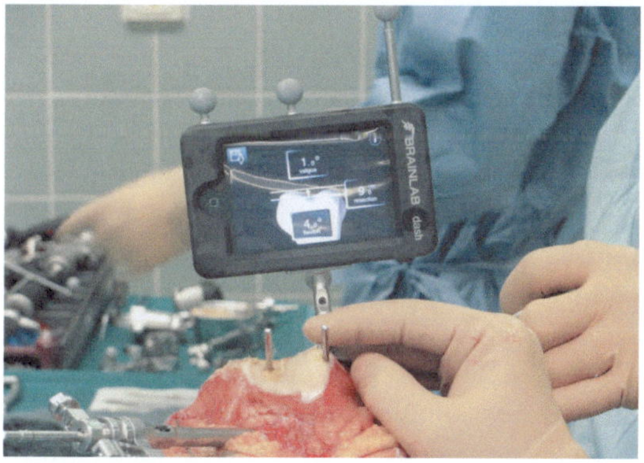

■ **Fig. 10.8** Verification of distal femur resection

This concept of presenting the information in line with the working field of the surgeon is in our opinion a major advantage of this new technology over existing navigation systems. Surgeons get instant visual feedback of their movements in the surgical field.

After the bone cut, the resection plane can be verified with the same technique and the results are saved for the final patient report.

The system is able to guide the distal femur and proximal tibia resection as well as the monitoring of the rotation alignment on the distal femur component based on a measured resection technique. In our personal experience, we prefer to align the femoral rotation using the conventional instruments either with a bony reference or a ligament-balanced technique.

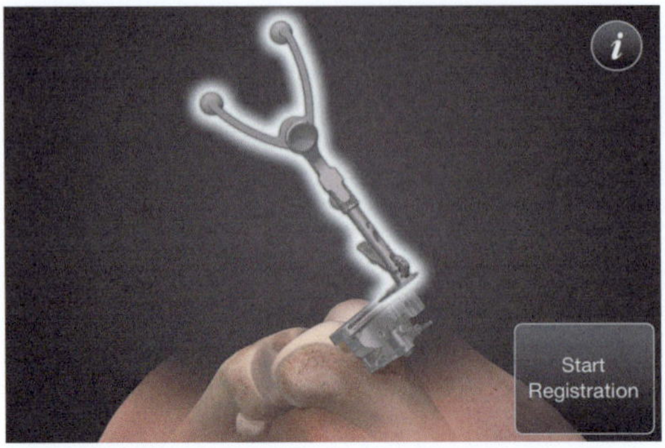

Fig. 10.9 Resection block with navigation array. (By courtesy of Brainlab AG)

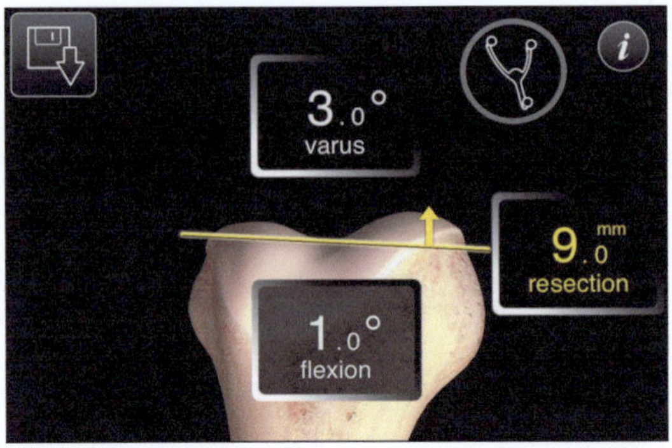

Fig. 10.10 Display of navigation results on the distal femur. (By courtesy of Brainlab AG)

10.1.7 Pinless Workflow for TKR

Available with version 1.1 of the software, a new »pinless workflow« was created for TKR software. This workflow met a major request of navigation users: to use the navigation technique without needing to fix static reference arrays to the femur and tibia. It was the aim of this development to create a highly time-saving procedure without compromising the precision of the navigation technique.

Within this workflow, the Dash® system can be used for navigation-assisted placement of the resection guides and for cut verification at the proximal tibia and distal femur both in primary as well as in revision TKR cases.

The resection guide in this workflow is placed in a preliminary resection position using either the conventional instruments or a fine-tunable cutting block. Without any additional arrangement, four landmarks have to be digitized to acquire the accurate three-dimensional position of the cutting block (Fig. 10.9).

This position together with the resection level, the varus/valgus alignment, and the extension/flexion position is displayed on the iPod® instantly (Fig. 10.10). For verification of the performed resection plane, only two landmarks have to be acquired. These data are stored for the final patient report. Because during surgery no additional reference arrays and landmark digitalizations are necessary, this workflow offers enormous improvements in the OR time required and reduces the complexity of the technique.

10.2 Clinical Experience

We started using the system as a prototype between August and December 2010 in 20 cases of total hip and knee replacement. This first clinical prototype study was approved by the German Federal Institute for Drugs and Medical Devices and the local ethics committee. The aim of this study was to evaluate the usability of the new Dash® concept in real joint replacement surgeries.

Usability was evaluated by different subjective and objective usability criteria and by time measurements of the different steps of the surgery and navigation process.

Many of the proposed advantages could already be demonstrated during these first clinical cases. The system showed the expected high grade of clinical usability by offering a short set-up time, clear and understandable workflow, and efficient integration into the surgery. This was even the case with new OR staff and assistants in each case. The scrub nurses were able to intuitively control the iPod® without special training. In this first series, procedures were performed between 1:06 h and 1:23 h for TKR and between 1:04 h and 1:58 h for THR, respectively, including one revision and several technical review cases. The additional time measured for the navigation period was an average 9 min for the hip surgery and the navigation/bone resection period was on average 13 min for the knee surgery. Even if it was not a primary objective of this study, the final leg alignment of the postoperative routine long leg standing radiographs showed an alignment within the safe corridor of ±3° varus/valgus in all TKR cases. Several technical improvements were identified in this clinical study, which were implemented into the final released system.

From October 2011, the Dash® system is now regularly used in our department primary and revision TKR and THR surgeries. The system has been used in about 110 computer-assisted joint replacement procedures. All cases are followed up with routine pre- and postoperative log leg standing radiographs or pelvic plain radiographs, respectively. The preliminary analysis of leg alignment and implant position data for the TKR procedures show equivalent results compared to previous published results with the Brainlab VectorVision® system, which is based on the same software calculations. These data represent leg alignment postoperatively in the upper 90% section within the safe zone of ±3°.

For the THR cases, we additionally found a high concordance between the hip geometry differences measured intraoperatively by the navigation system and the radiography measurement. Nevertheless, it should be clarified that the comparison of hip geometry on plain radiographs has its technical limitations. The final results of this data analysis will be published soon.

10.3 Discussion

Computer navigation in joint replacement surgery has developed into a very precise technique for intraoperatively optimized bone resection and implant positioning and also into a supporting technique for ligament-balancing procedures. The superior precision in creating a perfect leg alignment and implant position has been proven by numerous clinical studies even in routine clinical use in high caseload hospitals (Tingart et al. 2008). These data have been subject to several meta-analysis (Cheng et al. 2012). The navigation technique has met the primary goal of increased surgical precision.

Nevertheless, the technique is still far from being the standard of care in most countries. The technique now also competes with patient-specific resection guides that are produced preoperatively on the basis of an individual magnetic resonance imaging or computed tomography scan.

Besides the additional costs that are associated with the navigation technique, the complexity of the systems that are currently available has been identified as a major factor for not using this technique routinely.

Therefore, the Dash® system was designed especially to create a simple, smart, noncomplex navigation tool to address a larger community of surgeons.

According to the present experience of using the system in numerous routine primary and revision cases, we have been able to demonstrate that this concept of a commercial handheld iPod®-based navigation system is able to increase the acceptance of the navigation technique by both surgeons and by the whole surgical team.

10.4 Conclusion

Utilizing a revolutionary user interface technique with an iPod touch®, the Dash® system is a major forward in the wider usability and acceptance of the navigation technology in joint replacement surgery. The system enables a high-precision surgical technique without compromising the surgeon's workflow.

References

Cheng T, Zhao S, Peng X, Zhang X (2012) Does computer-assisted surgery improve postoperative leg alignment and implant positioning following total knee arthroplasty? A meta-analysis of randomized controlled trials? Knee Surg Sports Traumatol Arthrosc 20:1307–1322

Tingart M, Lüring C, Bäthis H, Beckmann J, Grifka J, Perlick L (2008) Computer-assisted total knee arthroplasty versus the conventional technique: how precise is navigation in clinical routine? Knee Surg Sports Traumatol Arthrosc 16:44–50

Benefits of Imageless Computer Navigation in Total Knee Arthroplasty

Christoph Schnurr, Dietmar Pierre König

Imageless computer navigation was introduced as a standard implantation technique for total knee arthroplasties (TKAs) more than a decade ago. According to arthroplasty registers, 11% of all TKAs in Western Australia, 2% in the United Kingdom, 19% in Norway, and 0.7% in Sweden have been implanted by use of computer navigation. These regional distinctions show that the debate over whether navigation is a feasible technique is still in progress.

This chapter intends to give an overview of the current literature and our own results concerning the proposed benefits of computer navigation. The effect of computer navigation on implant alignment, revision rate, and blood loss will be discussed.

11.1 Influence of Imageless Computer Navigation on Implant Alignment

Computer navigation was introduced in total knee arthroplasty (TKA) mainly to enable a more accurate placement of the prostheses and to avoid alignment outliers. In the following years, many studies focused on the alignment of navigated and conventional TKAs. To date, several meta-analyses have been published that compare both techniques. These studies are shown in ▫ Tab. 11.1.

For rating of the prosthesis alignment, studies have distinguished between alignment outliers, which differ more than 3° varus or valgus from the neutral mechanical axis, and the prosthesis within the 3° varus to 3° valgus corridor. While four of these studies included imageless and also a few image-guided navigation systems (Bäthis et al. 2006; Mason et al. 2007; Hetaimish et al. 2012; Fu et al. 2011; Bauwens et al. 2007), others included only imageless navigation devices (Brin et al. 2011). To summarize, regarding mechanical leg axis, all of the above-mentioned meta-analyses showed a significantly reduced rate of alignment outliers if navigation was used (▫ Fig. 11.1a,b). However, these studies did not focus only on the mechanical leg axis; some analyzed the three-dimensional implant alignment of the femoral and tibial component in detail (Mason et al. 2007; Brin et al. 2011; Hetaimish et al. 2012). These authors found a reduced rate of alignment outliers also in the coronal and sagittal plane if navigation was used. In conclusion, the meta-analyses show concordantly a significantly reduced rate of alignment outliers with the use of computer navigation. This was proven not only for the mechanical leg axis, but also for the three-dimensional implant alignment.

11.2 Influence of Computer Navigation on TKA Revision Rates

As mentioned, the discussion over navigated knee arthroplasty is still in progress. Advocates of the conventional, mechanical alignment technique argue against the longer operation times, elevated costs (Fang et al. 2009), the higher risks of fractures, and the missing long-term data for the navigated technique. By contrast, proponents of the navigated technique refer to the above-mentioned meta-ana-

▫ **Tab. 11.1** Overview of meta-analyses of alignment and computer navigation

Reference	Number of TKAs included		Outliers of >3° varus or valgus (%)	
	Conventional	Navigation	Conventional	Navigation
Bäthis et al. 2006	1,081	1,136	24%	6%
Mason et al. 2007	1,692	1,745	32%	9%
Brin et al. 2011	2,039	2,160	19%	4%
Hetaimish et al. 2012	1,302	1,374	30%	13%
Fu et al. 2011	1,020	1,119	29%	12%
Bauwens et al. 2007	1,716	1,707	n.a.	n.a.

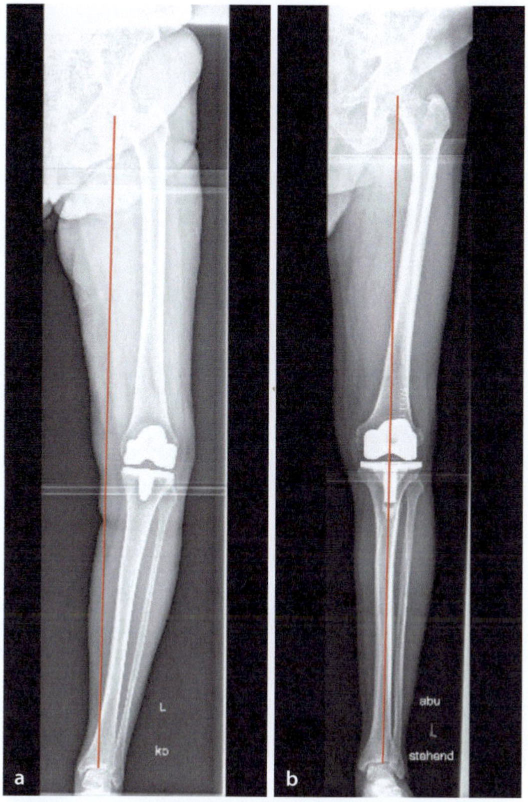

Fig. 11.1a,b **a** A patient who received a conventionally implanted TKA, resulting in varus misalignment. The *red line* represents the Mikulicz line. **b** A navigated TKA with a neutral mechanical leg axis

lyses that report on better postoperative alignment with navigation. Although the outcome of TKAs is multifactorial, it is generally assumed that restoration of the patient's normal mechanical axis is of paramount importance (Fang et al. 2009). This assumption is mainly based on studies that identified higher revision rates for alignment outliers (Fang et al. 2009; Ritter et al. 1994; Berend et al. 2004). Since a reduced risk of alignment outliers has been proven for navigated operations, advocates of the navigated procedure expect lower revision rates for navigated TKAs (Mullaji and Shetty 2009; Bäthis et al. 2006). In summary, the crux of the argument between proponents and critics of computer navigation is the potentially reduced revision rate, which might outweigh the higher costs of the procedure. Surprisingly, to date only very few studies have analyzed revision rates after conventional and navigated TKAs: Most of them focused on postoperative function and included fewer than 100 patients (Khan et al. 2012; Lutzner et al. 2010). These studies did not present any revision rates. Other studies included revision rates of navigated TKAs: Hernández-Vaquero et al. (2011) studied 100 patients with a follow-up of 8 years and detected similar revision rates between conventional and navigated techniques. Harvie et al. (2011) included 71 patients and found no revisions after 5 years. Pang et al. (2011) looked at 140 patients and found no revisions after 2 years, while Ishida studied 54 patients and had one revision in each group after 5 years (Ishida et al. 2011). Lüring et al. (2012) performed a matched-pair analysis of 100 patients and detected no revision after 5–7 years. In a recently published study, Hoffart et al. (2012) compared 5-year results after 97 conventional and 98 navigated TKAs. They found one revision in each group; however, follow-up was complete in only 62% of the patients. Besides these single-unit studies, data from the Norwegian arthroplasty register have been published (Gothesen et al. 2011). The authors included 1,465 navigated and 8,214 conventional TKAs with a mean follow-up of 1.4 years in the navigated group and 1.8 years in the conventional group. Their statistical analysis resulted in higher revisions rates for the navigated procedure than for the conventional TKAs (cumulative revisions rate at 2 years: navigated 3.6%, conventional 2.1%). In our own study, we compared the 1- to 6-year revision rates of 779 navigated and 342 conventional primary TKAs (Schnurr et al. 2012). In our study, 32 revisions were detected. In contrast to the Norwegian study, we found lower revision rates when computer navigation was used (Fig. 11.2, Cox proportional hazard model: $p=0.012$).

To allow further interpretation of our results, we analyzed the causes of revision in detail. In our study, the decreased revision rate for navigated operations was a result of the significantly lower rate of aseptic implant loosening (conventional TKAs 1.9%, navigated TKAs 0.1%, $p=0.024$) and a trend toward fewer joint instabilities (conventional TKAs 1.9%, navigated TKAs 1%, $p=0.439$).

To date, no long-term data comparing navigated and conventional TKAs have been published. The

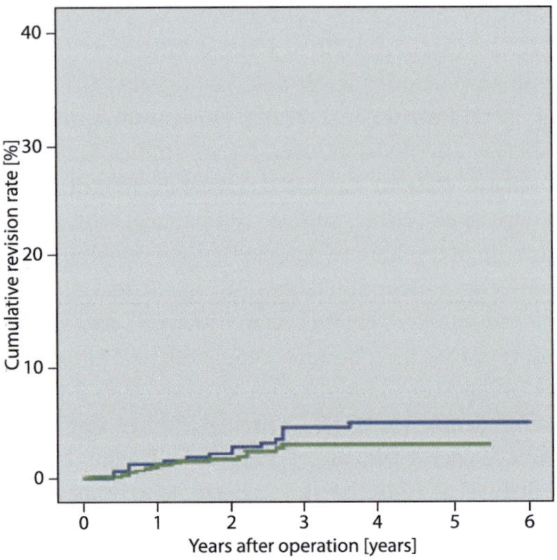

Fig. 11.2 Our study found significantly lower revision rates for navigated knee arthroplasties (*green line*) in comparison to conventionally implanted prostheses (*blue line*)

studies that include midterm revision rates yielded contradictory results. Therefore, it must be concluded that the published data are insufficient to evaluate the effect of computer navigation on the revision rates of TKAs.

11.3 Blood Loss

In the perioperative phase of TKA implantation, substantial blood loss is common. The anemia caused by this blood loss was generally identified as a perioperative risk factor. Therefore, allogenic blood transfusions are frequently required to avoid cardiovascular complications. However, the potential health risks associated with allogeneic blood include the transmission of blood-borne infections such as human immunodeficiency virus, hepatitis, transfusion-related and allergic reactions, and immunomodulatory effects. Moreover, blood transfusions are an additional cost for hospitals and health insurances. Therefore, efforts should be made to reduce the amount of blood loss and the need for blood transfusions in TKA. Effective methods to reduce blood loss and transfusion rates include the use of a tourniquet, minimally invasive surgery, and sealing of the intramedullary femoral canal.

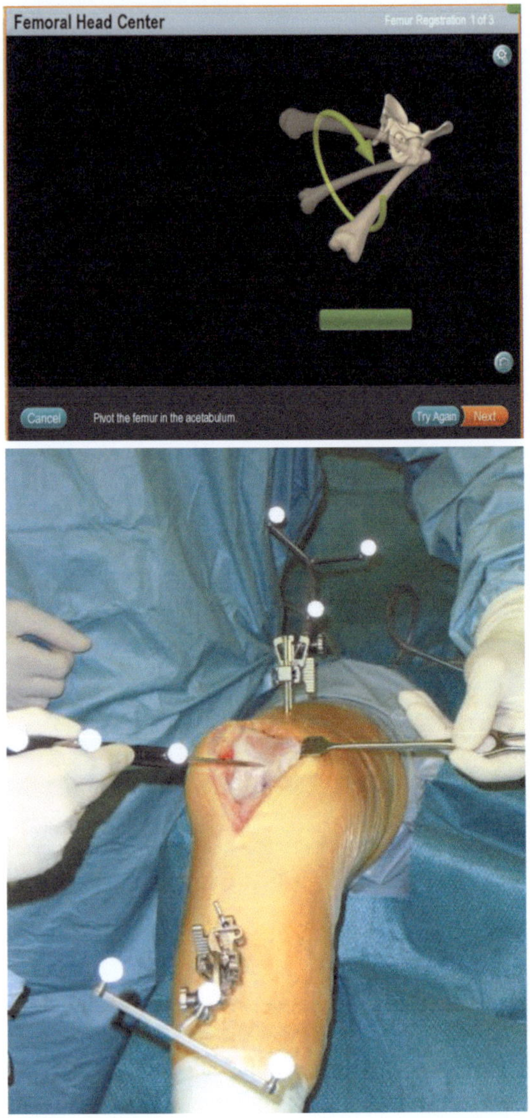

a

b

Fig. 11.3a,b The mechanical femoral axis is calculated by kinematic analysis of the hip rotational center (**a**) and the mechanical center of the distal femur (**b**)

Standard jig instruments for TKA require an opening of the femoral intramedullary canal to adjust the femoral component. This operative step has been identified as one of the reasons of the elevated blood loss and transfusion rate in TKA patients (Kandel et al. 2006). If computer navigation is used, the opening of the femoral medullary canal is not required: the femoral mechanical axis is calculated by kinematic analysis of the hip rotational center (Fig. 11.3a) and by referencing the mechanical center at the distal femur (Fig. 11.3b). Similarly, the tibia axis is calculated by identifying the tips of the ankle and the center of the tibial plateau.

Therefore, it seems logical that the use of imageless computer navigation might be an attractive option for diminishing blood loss. However, if post-surgery blood loss is to be compared between conventional and navigated techniques, the exclusive analysis of blood loss in wound drainages is inadequate. Studies have shown that the volume of the drainages represents only part of the total blood loss: There is 38–50% hidden blood loss after TKA. The hidden blood loss includes extravasation into the tissue, residual blood in the joint, and loss due to hemolysis. The total blood loss, including apparent blood loss in the drainages and hidden blood loss, can be calculated, for example, by the well-established OSTHEO formula (Rosencher et al. 2003).

To answer the question of whether navigation might diminish blood loss after TKA, we scanned the current literature for studies that analyzed total blood loss after conventional and navigated TKAs. We identified five studies including one of our own publications that met the above-mentioned criteria. Two additional studies were found that compared transfusion rates between conventional and navigated techniques. These data are shown in Tab. 11.2. To summarize, all studies identified lower blood loss for navigated TKAs than for conventionally aligned prostheses. The reduction of blood loss was significant in four of the five studies; Hinarejos et al. (2002) identified a trend toward lower blood loss for navigation, but it did not reach a level of significance.

Transfusion rates in conventional and in navigated TKAs were reported in four of these studies. A comparison between these studies is difficult to make because each used different surgical set-ups, tourniquets, and transfusion regimes. However, all the studies showed lower transfusion rates for navigated procedures, even if our study was the only one that found significant differences.

In this context, a study analyzed the data from the U.S. Nationwide Inpatient Sample Database (Browne et al. 2010). This database contains data of 101,596 TKAs, of which 1,156 were implanted by use of computer navigation. The authors identified fewer hematomas and a significantly reduced rate of postoperative cardiac complications when navigation was used.

In summary, all the available studies on total blood loss and transfusion rates have identified reduced blood loss and a trend toward fewer blood transfusions for navigated TKAs. However, it must be mentioned that to date only few studies exist and, therefore, data interpretation remains problematic.

Tab. 11.2 Studies on total blood loss or transfusion rate after TKA

Reference	Number of patients	Total blood loss (ml)		Transfusions (% of patients)	
		Conventional	Navigation	Conventional	Navigation
Kalairajah et al. (2005)	60	1,747	1,351*	–	–
Conteduca et al. (2009)	100	1,974	1,667*	–	–
Hinarejos et al. (2009)	87	750	712	23%	9%
Martin et al. (2007)	200	–	–	44%	38%
Millar et al. (2011)	61	1,399	1,105*	20%	13%
Schnurr et al. (2010)	447	1,375	1,242*	0.23/patient 15%	0.12/patient* 10%

* Significant differences

References

Bäthis H, Shafizadeh S, Paffrath T, Simanski C, Grifka J, Luring C (2006) Are computer assisted total knee replacements more accurately placed? A meta-analysis of comparative studies (in German). Orthopäde 35:1056–1065

Berend ME, Ritter MA, Meding JB, Faris PM, Keating EM, Redelman R, Faris GW, Davis KE (2004) Tibial component failure mechanisms in total knee arthroplasty. ClinOrthop Relat Res 428:26–34

Bauwens K, Matthes G, Wich M, Gebhard F, Hanson B, Ekkernkamp A, Stengel D (2007) Navigated total knee replacement. A meta-analysis. J Bone Joint Surg Am 89:261–269

Brin YS, Nikolaou VS, Joseph L, Zukor DJ, Antoniou J (2011) Imageless computer assisted versus conventional total knee replacement. A Bayesian meta-analysis of 23 comparative studies. Int Orthop 35:331–339

Browne JA, Cook C, Hofmann AA, Bolognesi MP (2010) Postoperative morbidity and mortality following total knee arthroplasty with computer navigation. Knee 17:152–156

Conteduca F, Massai F, Iorio R, Zanzotto E, Luzon D, Ferretti A (2009) Blood loss in computer-assisted mobile bearing total knee arthroplasty. A comparison of computer-assisted surgery with a conventional technique. Int Orthop 33:1609–1613

Fang DM, Ritter MA, Davis KE (2009) Coronal alignment in total knee arthroplasty: just how important is it? J Arthroplasty 24 [6 Suppl]:39–43

Fu Y, Wang M, Liu Y, Fu Q (2011) Alignment outcomes in navigated total knee arthroplasty: a meta-analysis. Knee Surg Sports Traumatol Arthrosc 20:1075–1082

Gothesen O, Espehaug B, Havelin L, Petursson G, Furnes O (2011) Short-term outcome of 1,465 computer-navigated primary total knee replacements 2005-2008. Acta Orthop 82:293–300

Harvie P, Sloan K, Beaver RJ (2011) Computer Navigation vs Conventional Total Knee Arthroplasty Five-Year Functional Results of a Prospective Randomized Trial. J Arthroplasty 27:667–672

Hernandez-Vaquero D, Suarez-Vazquez A, Iglesias-Fernandez S (2011) Can computer assistance improve the clinical and functional scores in total knee arthroplasty? Clin Orthop Relat Res 469:3436–3442

Hetaimish BM, Khan MM, Simunovic N, Al-Harbi HH, Bhandari M, Zalzal PK (2012) Meta-Analysis of navigation vs conventional total knee arthroplasty. J Arthroplasty 27:1177–1182

Hinarejos P, Corrales M, Matamalas A, Bisbe E, Caceres E (2009) Computer-assisted surgery can reduce blood loss after total knee arthroplasty. Knee Surg Sports Traumatol Arthrosc 17:356–360

Hoffart HE, Langenstein E, Vasak N (2012) A prospective study comparing the functional outcome of computer-assisted and conventional total knee replacement. Bone Joint Surg Br 94:194–199

Ishida K, Matsumoto T, Tsumura N, Kubo S, Kitagawa A, Chin T, Iguchi T, Kurosaka M, Kuroda R (2011) Mid-term outcomes of computer-assisted total knee arthroplasty. Knee Surg Sports Traumatol Arthrosc 19:1107–1112

Kalairajah Y, Simpson D, Cossey AJ, Verrall GM, Spriggins AJ (2005) Blood loss after total knee replacement: effects of computer-assisted surgery. J Bone Joint Surg Br 87:1480–1482

Kandel L, Vasili C, Kirsh G (2006) Extramedullary femoral alignment instrumentation reduces blood loss after uncemented total knee arthroplasty. J Knee Surg 19:256–258

Khan MM, Khan MW, Al-Harbi HH, Weening BS, Zalzal PK (2012) Assessing short-term functional outcomes and knee alignment of computer-assisted navigated total knee arthroplasty. J Arthroplasty 27:271–277

Luring C, Kauper M, Bathis H, Perlick L, Beckmann J, Grifka J, Tingart M, Rath B (2012) A five to seven year follow-up comparing computer-assisted vs freehand TKR with regard to clinical parameters. Int Orthop 36:553–558

Lutzner J, Gunther KP, Kirschner S (2010) Functional outcome after computer-assisted versus conventional total knee arthroplasty: a randomized controlled study. Knee Surg Sports Traumatol Arthrosc 18:1339–1344

Martin A, Wohlgenannt O, Prenn M, Oelsch C, von SA (2007) Imageless navigation for TKA increases implantation accuracy. Clin Orthop Relat Res 460:178–184

Mason JB, Fehring TK, Estok R, Banel D, Fahrbach K (2007) Meta-analysis of alignment outcomes in computer-assisted total knee arthroplasty surgery. J Arthroplasty 22:1097–1106

Millar NL, Deakin AH, Millar LL, Kinnimonth AW, Picard F (2011) Blood loss following total knee replacement in the morbidly obese: Effects of computer navigation. Knee 18:108–112

Mullaji A, Shetty GM (2009) Computer-assisted TKA: greater precision, doubtful clinical efficacy: opposes. Orthopedics 32:25

Pang HN, Yeo SJ, Chong HC, Chin PL, Ong J, Lo NN (2011) Computer-assisted gap balancing technique improves outcome in total knee arthroplasty, compared with conventional measured resection technique. Knee Surg Sports Traumatol Arthrosc 19:1496–1503

Ritter MA, Faris PM, Keating EM, Meding JB (1994) Postoperative alignment of total knee replacement. Its effect on survival. Clin Orthop Relat Res 299:153–156

Rosencher N, Kerkkamp HE, Macheras G, Munuera LM, Menichella G, Barton DM, Cremers S, Abraham IL (2003) Orthopedic Surgery Transfusion Hemoglobin European Overview (OSTHEO) study: blood management in elective knee and hip arthroplasty in Europe. Transfusion 43:459–469

Schnurr C, Csecsei G, Eysel P, Konig DP (2010) The Effect of Computer Navigation on Blood Loss and Transfusion Rate in TKA. Orthopedics 33:10–08

Schnurr C, Güdden I, Eysel P, König DP (2012) Influence of computer navigation on TKAs revision rate. Int Orthop 36:2255–2260

Renaissance of Robotics in TKA

The Mako Robotic System for Unicompartmental Knee Arthroplasty

Mustafa Citak, Andrew D. Pearle, Daniel O. Kendoff

Robotic systems have been used in surgery since 1980, while the integration of robotic systems in orthopedic surgery began with the use of RoboDoc (Curexo Technology Corporation, Fremont, CA, USA) for the planning and performing of robotic-assisted total hip arthroplasty (THA) in 1992. The use of robotic technology has facilitated minimally invasive surgery in some cases, which has gained popularity in patients (Banks 2009). Another advantage of robotic surgery is the higher precision and accuracy compared to conventional techniques, which is of enormous importance especially in spinal surgery (Devito et al. 2010). Current robotic systems can be classified as autonomous, haptic, surgeon-guided systems. Haptic or surgeon-guided robotic systems allow the surgeon to use the robot to perform the surgery. The permanent input of the surgeon is mandatory to perform the procedure. By contrast, in autonomous systems, the surgeon performs the approach and set-up of the system and then engages the robot to finish the surgery without the surgeon's help. A historical example of autonomous systems is RoboDoc (RoboDoc, Sacramento, CA, USA), which was especially popular in Germany in the 1990s. Statistically significant higher accuracy in implant positioning has been reported with the use of RoboDoc compared to conventional systems (Bargar 2007). However, nowadays, owing to the higher complication rate and safety concerns, the use of RoboDoc has sharply declined (Davies et al. 2007; Schulz et al. 2007). Nevertheless, the use of robotic systems has recently increased, especially the use of haptic or surgeon-guided systems.

12.1 Unicompartmental Knee Arthroplasty with Haptic Robotic Systems

Unicompartmental knee arthroplasty (UKA) was introduced in the early 1970s and today is commonly used for the treatment of isolated compartmental osteoarthritis of the knee (Berger et al. 1999; Suggs et al. 2006). UKA did not gain wide acceptance because of the high failure rate and poor outcome (Insall and Aglietti 1980). However, recent improvements in implant design, minimally invasive techniques, bone-sparing strategies, expanded indications, and early rehabilitation have all contributed to a renewed enthusiasm for UKA.

UKA has been shown to be a good and less-invasive alternative to total knee arthroplasty (TKA), especially for younger and active patients (Ohdera et al. 2001). Advantages of UKA include better postoperative range of motion, less soft tissue dissection, preservation of bone stock, minimal blood loss, faster recovery, lower complication rates, and more physiological function (Ohdera et al. 2001; Koskinen et al. 2009).

Nevertheless, early failures of femoral and tibial components have also been reported (Berend et al. 2005; Collier et al. 2006; Furnes et al. 2007; Mariani et al. 2007). Failures attributed to overcorrection and undercorrection have received the most attention (Hernigou and Deschamps 2004a, 2004b; Jeer et al. 2004; Ridgeway et al. 2002).

The use of computer-assisted surgery systems in UKA has resulted in improved postoperative alignment, reduction of outliers, and better postoperative clinical results (Buckup et al. 2007; Molfetta and Caldo 2008; Haaker et al. 2006). Cobb and colleagues (2006) reported that robot-assisted placement of UKA (Acrobot Sculptor; Acrobot Company, Ltd., London, UK) components was more accurate than traditional techniques and that, subsequently, clinical outcomes were improved. Cobb's method, however, employed rigid intraoperative stabilization of the bones in a stereotactic frame, which is impractical for routine clinical use.

The »Robotic Arm Interactive Orthopedic System« (RIO; MAKO Surgical Corp., Fort Lauderdale, FL, USA) (▪ Fig. 12.1), is an example of a surgeon-guided robotic system that allows for dynamic bone tracking, which is of enormous intraoperative importance.

12.2 Preoperative Imaging and Planning

Preoperative computed tomography (CT) scans are obtained using specific scan protocols for all patients. The CT data are saved in DICOM (Digital Imaging and Communications in Medicine; Rosslyn, VA, USA) format and transferred to the software of the robotic system (MAKO Surgical Corp.).

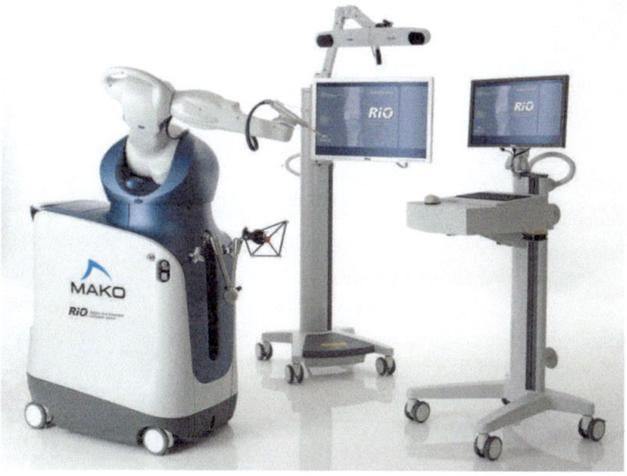

■ **Fig. 12.1** The »Robotic Arm Interactive Orthopedic System« (RIO) as an example of a surgeon-guided robotic system. (By courtesy of MAKO Surgical Corp.)

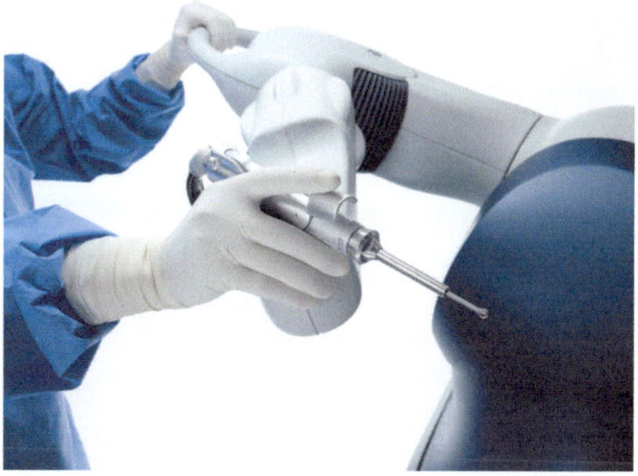

■ **Fig. 12.2** The high-frequency burr is equipped at the distal end of the robot. (By courtesy of MAKO Surgical Corp.)

The bone surfaces are segmented in the software to create a patient-specific three-dimensional (3D) model of the knee.

CT-based planning is ideal for bony alignment including the assessment of osteophyte formations, cysts, or necrosis. However, CT-based planning also has its limitations. For example, soft tissues cannot be visualized with CT.

On the basis of the preoperative CT scan, the system allows for preoperative planning of the femoral and tibial implant position including the following aspects:

- Alignment parameters and intraoperative gap kinematics
- 3D virtual visualization of implant position

After planning and defining the optimal implant position, the data are saved in the system, while the system automatically defines the boundaries of bony resection.

12.3 Intraoperative Set-up and Surgical Technique

Positioning of the robotic system is performed before the patient's arrival in the operating room (OR). The positioning of the system is based on the affected knee and the surgeon's dominant hand. The haptic or surgeon-guided system (MAKO Surgical Corp.) consists of three components: robotic arm, optical camera, and operator computer cart (■ Fig. 12.1). The distal end of the robotic arm is equipped with a high-speed bone-resecting burr (■ Fig. 12.2). After sterile draping of the patient's leg and performing a tissue-sparing exposure, reference optical arrays are placed into the distal femur and proximal tibia using Steinman pins and also mounted on the robotic arm. After a routine registration process, the robotic arm-assisted resection process of the planned femoral and tibial surface can be performed (■ Fig. 12.3). The surgeon moves the robotic arm by guiding the force-controlled tip within the defined boundaries. While inside the volume of bone to be resected, the robotic arm operates without offering any resistance. As the

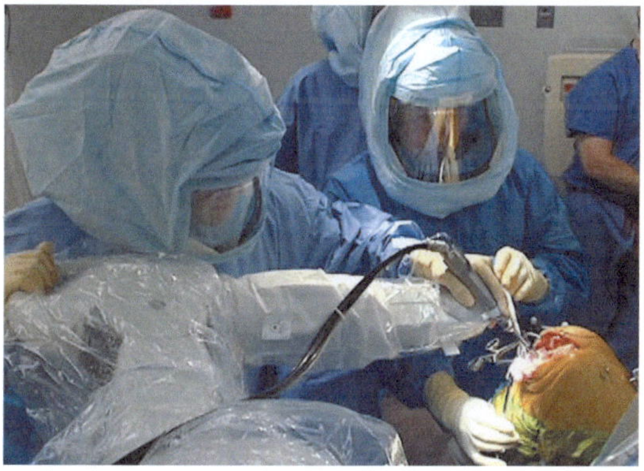

■ **Fig. 12.3** Intraoperative set-up of the MAKO system during a robotic-assisted unicompartmental knee arthroplasty. (By courtesy of MAKO Surgical Corp.)

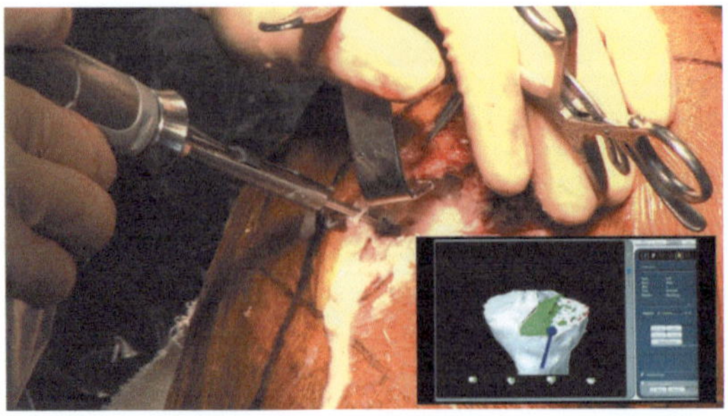

Fig. 12.4 Intraoperative image during a robotic-assisted unicompartmental knee arthroplasty. The *main image* shows the burring process of the femoral bone surface. The *inset* is a screenshot of the system showing the 3D visualization as a guide for the surgeon. (By courtesy of MAKO Surgical Corp.)

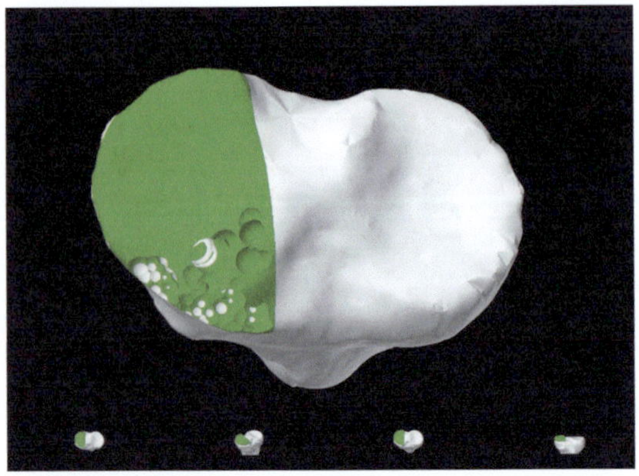

Fig. 12.5 Screenshot showing the 3D visualization of the planned tibial resection. The *green area* is a visual guide for the surgeon showing the area still to be resected. (By courtesy of MAKO Surgical Corp.)

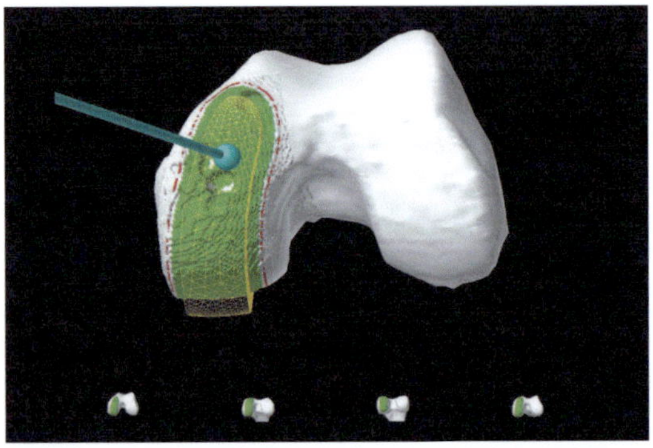

Fig. 12.6 The *green area* reveals the part of the femoral bone still to be resected. (By courtesy of MAKO Surgical Corp.)

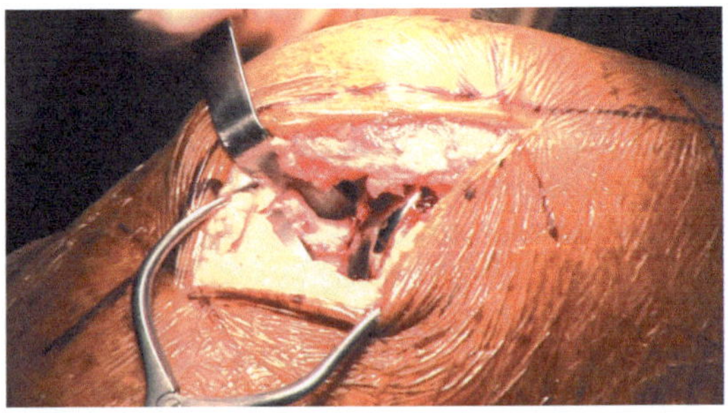

Fig. 12.7 Intraoperative situs showing the postoperative result after implantation of the prosthesis. (By courtesy of MAKO Surgical Corp.)

burr approaches the boundary, the robotic arm resists that motion and haptically keeps the burr within the accepted volume (Fig. 12.4).

It is recommended to perform first the tibial and then the femoral resection. However, the specific sequence can also be selected individually by the surgeon. Permanent visual feedback on the navigation screen shows the actually achieved versus the planned resection, which is based on the preoperative planning (Fig. 12.5 and Fig. 12.6).

Once both compartments have been prepared, femoral and tibial component trials are inserted and a full flexion – extension arc can be performed. Computerized simulation of the implants reveals the actual overlapping of the implant components, giving the surgeon feedback about the actual leg alignment and knee gap kinematics.

After acceptance of the implant positioning, both components are cemented and a final analysis of the implant kinematics and limb alignment is made (Fig. 12.7). The reference arrays and mini-checkpoints are then removed and a standard wound closure is performed.

12.4 Outcomes of Robotic-Assisted Unicompartmental Knee Arthroplasty

The Acrobot® (acronym for Active Constraint Robot) system, another tactile system with several similarities to the RIO system, was introduced in 2001 (Jakopec et al. 2001). In a prospective randomized double-blind (patient and assessor) study,

Cobb et al. (2006) presented the results of robotic-assisted UKA using the Acrobot system compared to conventional UKA. A total of 27 patients were recruited in the study. In addition to the radiological differences in the planned and achieved tibiofemoral angles, the American Knee Society (AKS) score and Western Ontario and McMaster Universities osteoarthritis index (WOMAC) were evaluated in all patients. In the robotic group, all of the patients had tibiofemoral alignment in the coronal plane within 2° of the planned position. However, in only 40% of the conventional group was this level of accuracy achieved. There was also a significant difference in the AKS score between both groups, with a mean increase of the AKS score twice as large in the Acrobot system group. However, in the robotic-assisted group, an additional operative time of 16 min was required compared to the conventional technique. Another drawback of this system is the necessity of employing rigid intraoperative stabilization of the bones in a stereotactic frame. Robotic systems have now evolved to include dynamic bone-tracking technologies so that rigid fixation is no longer required.

Pearle et al. reported the first clinical series of ten implanted UKAs using a robotic system with dynamic bone-tracking technology (Pearle et al. 2010). No outliers or complications were noted in the study. The difference between the planned and the intraoperative tibiofemoral angle was less than 1° (Pearle et al. 2010).

Roche et al. (unpublished data) analyzed the first 43 robotic-assisted UKAs using radiographic measurements performed by an independent reviewer. Of the 344 radiographic measurements, only three femoral components were considered to be outliers. Hence, less than 1% of the measurements were found to be outliers (Sinha 2009).

Sinha and colleagues (2009) reported on their first 20 cases of robotic arm-assisted UKA. They concluded that robotically assisted UKA has extremely accurate bone preparation relative to the preoperative plan and is a reliably accurate tool.

In a recent study, Lonner et al. (2010) compared the postoperative radiographic alignment of the tibial component with the preoperatively planned position with and without the use of robotics and found a higher root mean square (RMS) error of the posterior tibial slope and a higher varus/valgus RMS error with the conventional technique.

Coon (2009) found that the RMS error of the posterior tibial slope was 2.5 times better, the variance was 2.8 times lower, and varus alignment 3.2° better in the robotic group compared to the conventional technique.

Based on an analysis of 223 robotic-assisted cases using the MAKO platform contributed from three centers, the complication rates and patient outcomes were also analyzed (Sinha 2009). In total, six revision surgeries (2.7%) were required because of infection (n=2), femoral shaft fracture (n=1), arthrofibrotic band release (n=1), arthrotomy dehiscence (n=1), and unexplained pain (n=1). Implant loosening, as a cause for revision surgery, was not reported in these series. Moreover, a postoperative statistically significant improvement in range of motion (ROM), Knee Society Score (KSS), WOMAC scores, pain and stiffness was shown in these patients.

Despite the described advantages of robotic systems, there are also disadvantages. These mainly include the high costs and longer surgery time. The required preoperative CT scan and preoperative planning increase the overall time, effort, and cost (Swank et al. 2009). Learning curve issues associated with new techniques should also be considered. However, the surgery time decreased after 20 cases from 80–120 min to 40 min after integration of the MAKO system into the operating room, as reported by Coon (2009).

12.5 Conclusion

The use of robotic technology offers promising short-term results compared to traditional conventional orthopedic procedures. The technological innovations and advances help the surgeon perform a more precise surgery with preoperative planning and robotic-assisted resection. However, financial barriers and the lack of long-term prospective studies are still limiting factors to the widespread use of robotic technology. Although the improved short-term results of lower blood loss and faster rehabilitation support the use of robotic technology, further studies are required to identify whether robotic technology truly improves the long-term outcome.

References

Banks SA (2009) Haptic robotics enable a systems approach to design of a minimally invasive modular knee arthroplasty. Am J Orthop (Belle Mead NJ) 38:23–27

Bargar WL (2007) Robots in orthopaedic surgery: past, present, and future. Clinl Orthop Relat Res 463:31–36

Berend KR, Lombardi AV Jr, Mallory TH, Adams JB, Groseth KL (2005) Early failure of minimally invasive unicompartmental knee arthroplasty is associated with obesity. Clin Orthop Relat Res 440:60–66

Berger RA, Nedeff DD, Barden RM et al (1999) Unicompartmental knee arthroplasty. Clinical experience at 6- to 10-year follow-up. Clin Orthop Relat Res 36750–60

Buckup K, Linke LC, Hahne V (2007) Minimally invasive implantation and computer navigation for a unicondylar knee system. Orthopedics 30:66–69

Cobb J, Henckel J, Gomes P et al (2006) Hands-on robotic unicompartmental knee replacement: a prospective, randomised controlled study of the acrobot system. J Bone Joint Surg Br 88:188–197

Collier MB, Eickmann TH, Sukezaki F, McAuley JP, Engh GA (2006) Patient, implant, and alignment factors associated with revision of medial compartment unicondylar arthroplasty. J Arthroplasty 21:108–115

Coon TM (2009) Integrating robotic technology into the operating room. Am J Orthop (Belle Mead NJ) 38:7–9

Davies BL, Rodriguez y Baena FM, Barrett AR et al (2007) Robotic control in knee joint replacement surgery. Proceedings of the Institution of Mechanical Engineers Part H. J Eng Med 221:71–80

Devito DP, Kaplan L, Dietl R et al (2010) Clinical acceptance and accuracy assessment of spinal implants guided with SpineAssist surgical robot: retrospective study. Spine 35:2109–2115

Furnes O, Espehaug B, Lie SA, et al (2007) Failure mechanisms after unicompartmental and tricompartmental primary knee replacement with cement. J Bone Joint Surg Am 89:519–525

Haaker RG, Wojciechowski M, Patzer P, Willburger RE, Senkal M, Engelhardt M (2006) Minimally invasive unicondylar knee placement with computer navigation. Orthopaede 34:1073–1079

Hernigou P, Deschamps G (2004a) Alignment influences wear in the knee after medial unicompartmental arthroplasty. Clin Orthop Relat Res 423:161–165

Hernigou P, Deschamps G (2004b) Posterior slope of the tibial implant and the outcome of unicompartmental knee arthroplasty. J Bone Joint Surg Am 86:506-511

Insall J, Aglietti P (1980) A five to seven-year follow-up of unicondylar arthroplasty. J Bone Joint Surg 62:1329–1337

Jakopec M, Harris SJ, Rodriguez y Baena F et al (2001) The first clinical application of a »hands-on« robotic knee surgery system. Comput Aided Surg 6:329–339

Jeer PJ, Keene GC, Gill P (2004) Unicompartmental knee arthroplasty: an intermediate report of survivorship after the introduction of a new system with analysis of failures. Knee 11:369–374

Koskinen E, Paavolainen P, Eskelinen A et al (2009) Medial unicompartmental knee arthroplasty with Miller-Galante II prosthesis: mid-term clinical and radiographic results. Arch Orthop Trauma Surg 2009;129:617–624

Lonner JH, John TK, Conditt MA (2010) Robotic arm-assisted UKA improves tibial component alignment: a pilot study. Clin Orthop Relat Res 468:141–146

Mariani EM, Bourne MH, Jackson RT, Jackson ST, Jones P (2007) Early failure of unicompartmental knee arthroplasty. J Arthroplasty 22:81–84

Molfetta L, Caldo D (2008) Computer navigation versus conventional implantation for varus knee total arthroplasty: a case-control study at 5 years follow-up. Knee 15:75–79

Ohdera T, Tokunaga J, Kobayashi A (2001) Unicompartmental knee arthroplasty for lateral gonarthrosis: midterm results. J Arthroplasty 16:196–200

Pearle AD, O'Loughlin PF, Kendoff DO (2010) Robot-assisted unicompartmental knee arthroplasty. J Arthroplasty 25:230–237

Ridgeway SR, McAuley JP, Ammeen DJ, Engh GA (2002) The effect of alignment of the knee on the outcome of unicompartmental knee replacement. J Bone Joint Surg 84:351–355

Schulz AP, Seide K, Queitsch C, et al (2007) Results of total hip replacement using the Robodoc surgical assistant system: clinical outcome and evaluation of complications for 97 procedures. MRCAS 3:301–306

Sinha RK (2009) Outcomes of robotic arm-assisted unicompartmental knee arthroplasty. Am J Orthop (Belle Mead NJ) 38:20–22

Suggs JF, Li G, Park SE et al (2006) Knee biomechanics after UKA and its relation to the ACL – a robotic investigation. J Orthop Res 24:588–594

Swank ML, Alkire M, Conditt M, Lonner JH (2009) Technology and cost-effectiveness in knee arthroplasty: computer navigation and robotics. Am J Orthop (Belle Mead NJ) 38:32–36

Innovation in the Navigation of THA

Hip Navigation Using the OrthoPilot® System

Thilo Floerkemeier; Henning Windhagen

Total hip arthroplasty (THA) is one of the most successful orthopedic surgeries performed worldwide. More than 200,000 THAs are implanted in Germany each year. Critical to the success of these surgeries is the accurate positioning of the components. The orientation of the cup positioning affects directly the success and survival of the THA and may have an influence on the patient's functional outcome.

13.1 Importance of Cup Positioning

Malpositioning of the implant components is the major cause for early joint dislocation, limited range of motion due to femoroacetabular impingement, and early implant wear due to edge loading and leg length discrepancies (Kennedy et al. 1998; McCollum and Gray 1990; Schmalzried et al. 1994; Turner 1994; Williamson and Reckling 1978) (■ Fig. 13.1). An increased anteversion or inclination of the cup may result in a higher risk of dislocation and mechanical wear due to edge loading (■ Fig. 13.2a,b). The consequence of malpositioning depends among other things on the bearing materials used. The risk of mechanical wear is increased with polyethylene inlays (■ Fig. 13.3). For modern hard-on-hard bearing surfaces, such as ceramic-on-ceramic and metal-on-metal, an exact orientation of the cup is important to prevent ceramic fracture, squeaking, or increased metal ion release in metal-on-metal bearings (Clarke et al. 2003; Gonzalez et al. 2011; Jacobs et al. 2003; Vendittoli et al. 2010). A decreased inclination and anteversion may lead to femoroacetabular impingement and thus to a limitation in range of motion. Therefore, new ways to improve the longevity of THA are becoming increasingly important.

The importance of cup orientation was mentioned by Lewinnek and colleagues as early as 1978. They defined a safe zone for cup orientation concerning inclination and anteversion to minimize the previously mentioned complications (inclination: 40°±10°; anteversion: 15°±10°) (Lewinnek et al. 1978). In a series of 300 total hip replacements, they determined a dislocation rate of 1.5% for cup positioning within the »safe zone« compared to 6.1% for cups positioned outside the safe zone. In addition, different studies report on a very high rate of revision (one third of all revisions) within the first 5 years after THA following recurrent dislocations (DiGioia III et al. 2003; Dobzyniak et al. 2006; Yuan and Shih 1999). Besides lowering the risk of complications, accurate positioning of the implants is important for reconstructing the offset, the limb length, and thus the biomechanics of the physiological hip. Recently, Widmer and Zurfluh introduced the concept of the »femur-first« method (Widmer and Zurfluh 2004). This concept of combined anteversion for THA proposes a relationship between the acetabular and femoral components that theoretically maximizes the postoperative range of motion and minimizes the risk for impingement of the joint. Using computer-assisted navigation tools, an anteversion angle of the cup component can be made to be dependent on the antetorsion angle of the stem component (or vice versa). Widmer proposed a combined anteversion of 37.3°, whereas the femoral antetorsion should be only 70% (anteversion of cup + 70% of antetorsion of the stem = 37.3°). Sendtner and coworkers conducted a prospective study on this concept and concluded that the combined anteversion concept results in a cup position with more anteversion when compared to the traditional cup placement according to the Lewinnek safe zone (Sendtner et al. 2010). In this context, they believe that modern navigation techniques open a new frontier for an optimized component position, because placing the acetabular and femoral component in relation to the anteversion for both compo-

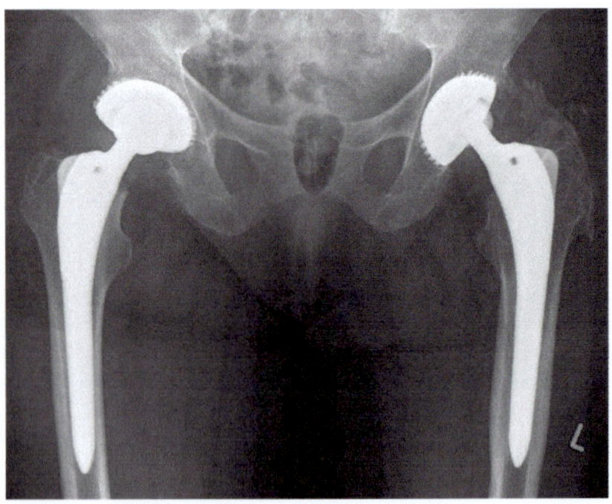

■ **Fig. 13.1** X-ray of a pelvis in anteroposterior view with different positioning of the cups: a small inclination of the right hip and a large inclination of the left hip

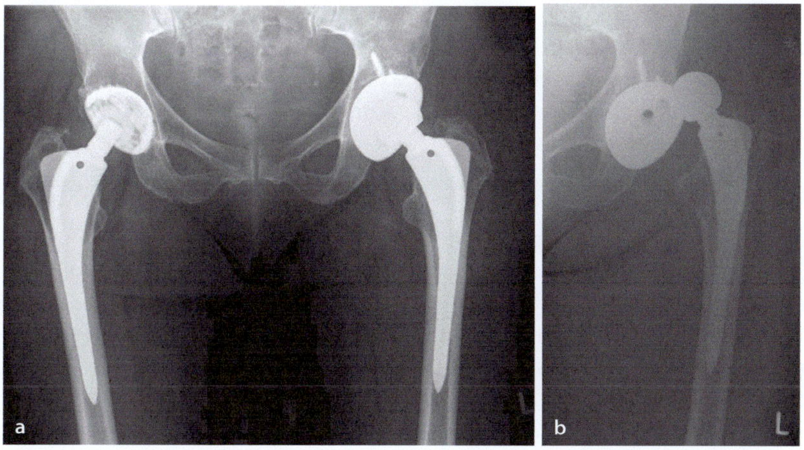

Fig. 13.2a,b X-ray of a pelvis in anteroposterior view with an increased inclination of the left cup (**a**) and the associated complication of hip dislocation (**b**)

nents allows patient-specific biomechanics to be considered.

13.2 Navigation for Correct Implant Orientation

Traditionally, correct component alignment depends on the surgeon referencing from the position of the patient on the table and the anatomical landmarks (Punwar et al. 2011). However, this may result in a wide variability in component positioning. Factors such as pelvic tilt are sometimes difficult to determine intraoperatively and they have an effect on cup positioning (Lin et al. 2011). Nishikubo and colleagues evaluated the preoperative errors in the pelvic tilt of 249 hips before THA using fluoroscopic imaging while the patients were in the lateral decubitus position (Nishikubo et al. 2011). The mean absolute value errors of the pelvic tilt were 2.94° (SD, 2.92°), 2.49° (SD, 2.68°), and 5.92° (SD, 5.20°) in the coronal, transverse, and sagittal planes, respectively. Thus, they regard such preoperative errors in the pelvic tilt as contributing to malpositioning of the acetabular component, since it is frequently observed on postoperative radiographs. Furthermore, in case of congenital deformities or deviations in anatomy due to previous reorientation surgery, as in patients with dysplasia, the intraoperative orientation according to anatomic landmarks may be misleading. Therefore, intraoperative radiography is one option for confirming the correct positioning of the components.

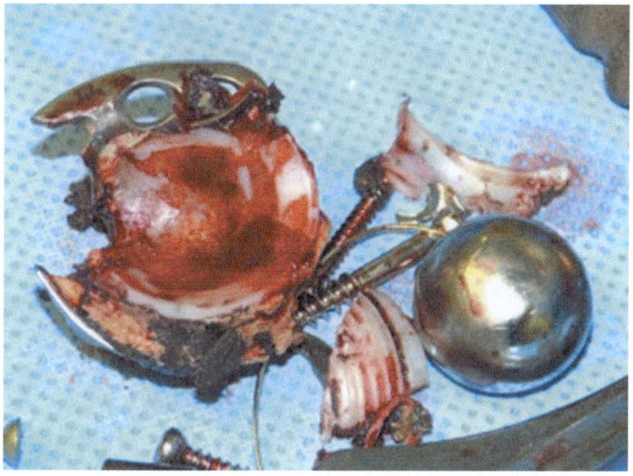

Fig. 13.3 Wear and destruction of a polyethylene inlay and a revision cup as a possible complication of edge loading

Navigation represents an alternative tool for this task. Computer navigation systems were introduced in the past to provide surgeons with data on acetabular and femoral positioning so that leg length, femoral offset, and range of motion are determined before the definite implantation of the components (Dastane et al. 2011). The surgeon is able to view lines, angles, and measurements for the implantation of THA in order to align and orient the components more precisely. Thus, navigation assists and optimizes cup positioning and simultaneously avoids radiation exposure. Two different concepts of navigation exist: image-based navigation and image-free navigation. Image-based navigation is based on a preoperative computed tomography scan. This concept has advantages for patients with anatomic deformities, such as coxarthrosis due to dysplasia or trauma. However, it is associated with a high radiation exposure. Because of this and the higher expenditures regarding time and money, today image-free navigation represents the gold standard. In the past, many companies developed mechanical guides for cup and stem positioning such as the OrthoPilot® (Aesculap Orthopaedics, Tuttlingen, Germany) as a tool for the precise execution of surgical interventions. OrthoPilot® is a computer-aided, image-free navigation system. The navigation system consists of infrared optics and tracking software continually monitoring the position and mechanical alignment of the components relative to the patient's individual anatomy. Minimally invasive smart wireless instruments send data to a computer, which analyzes these data and provides the angles, lines, and measurements needed to best align the components of the THA. The surgeon is able to change the positioning in real time. OrthoPilot® uses passive trackers to register the orientation of the pelvis intraoperatively with the registration of bony landmarks. Definition of the bony landmarks is important for the final accuracy of the positioning (Parratte and Argenson 2007; Renkawitz et al. 2009). The first experiments in kinematic navigation using OrthoPilot® were conducted as early as 1994. In the following years, further developments took place and a multicenter study was conducted (Aesculap 2012). The first clinical application and first publication dates back to 1997. Since its introduction in the market in 2001, more than 15,000 THAs have been implanted using this device.

13.3 Evidence of Benefits Using Navigation

In the last decade there was a tendency toward minimally invasive or less invasive surgery. During these interventions there is often a limited view of the operative field, which often makes perfect implant positioning very complicated (DiGioia III et al. 2003; Nogler 2004). Especially in these cases, special tools or landmarks for component positioning, such as computer navigation technology, can support the surgeon despite the lack of direct visualization of anatomical landmarks (DiGioia III et al. 2002; Sotereanos et al. 2006). Gebel et al. analyzed their new concept of using the minimally invasive direct anterior approach (DAA) in total hip replacement (THR) in combination with a leg positioner (Rotex-table®) and a modified retractor system (Condor, Salzkotten, Germany). All surgeries were performed using hip navigation. Radiological analysis illustrated an average cup inclination of 43° and a leg length discrepancy in the range of ±5 mm in 99% of cases, showing the benefit of the navigation tool (Gebel et al. 2012). Confalonieri and coworkers performed a match-pair study between computer-assisted and freehand techniques using a short modular femoral stem (Confalonieri et al. 2008). They assessed surgical time, clinical outcome, dislocation rate, limb length, and offset in 44 patients and concluded that computer-assisted techniques allowed for easier management of limb length discrepancy and offset restoring. The postoperative leg length discrepancy was 4.1 mm for the navigated implantation and 7.9 mm for the conventional technique, while the preoperative leg length discrepancy was similar for both groups. In addition, Kreuzer and Leffers conducted a retrospective study comparing a consecutive series of 150 computer-navigated THAs with a consecutive series of 150 nonnavigated hips (Kreuzer and Leffers 2011). The two groups were similarly matched by age, gender, and body mass index. The navigation group mean cup inclination was 41° (range, 32°–54°), compared to 36° (range, 19°–52°) for the nonnavigated group. The authors concluded that the accuracy and precision of cup angle placement is comparable to the nonnavigated method but appears to be slightly improved with computer navigation. The high accuracy of the navigation tool was also confirmed in several other studies (Beckmann et al. 2009; Hohmann et al. 2011b, 2011c; Lin et al. 2011; Moskal and Capps 2011; Snyder et al. 2012). Snyder and colleagues evaluated the accuracy of a particular imageless computer navigation system in determining cup position (Snyder et al. 2012). After assessment of 39 patients, they determined a high specificity for navigation when assessing cup abduction and anteversion (specificity >90%). However, the system was not very effective in detecting suboptimal cup position (sensitivity: abduction, 50%; anteversion, 33%). Hohmann et al. compared acetabular component positioning using an imageless system with a matched control group using conventional techniques (Hohmann et al. 2011c). They demonstrated a significant increase in the accuracy of placement of acetabular cups within the desired position and safe zone using imageless navigation. In another study by Hohmann et al., the authors assessed and validated intraoperative placement values for both inclination and anteversion as displayed by an imageless navigation system compared to postoperative measurement of cup position using high-resolution CT scans (Hohmann et al. 2011b). Their findings determined a possible introduction of systematic error. Even though the acquisition of anatomic landmarks is simple, they must be acquired with great precision. An error of 1 cm can result in a mean anteversion error of 6° and an inclination error of 2.5°. Despite possible errors, navigation seems to offer a possible patient benefit from the resulting tighter control of the component position. This is also the conclusion of a meta-analysis reviewing published studies in order to investigate the claim of the increased precision of acetabular component placement in navigated THA compared to conventional, nonnavigated THA. In this review, 1,479 procedures were included. Moskal and Capps determined a statistically significant difference in the incidence of acetabular component placement in the »safe zone«, with navigation having significantly more »safe placements« than procedures without navigation, regardless of the chosen safe zone (Moskal and Capps 2011). In addition, navigated THAs had significantly fewer dislocations than nonnavigated THAs. Another meta-analysis published by Beckmann et al. confirmed navigation as being a reliable tool for optimizing cup placement and minimizing outliers (Beckmann et al. 2009).

A cadaveric study also determined a reduced variability in cup positioning for navigated versus manual THAs by measuring the inclination and anteversion using CT scans (Nogler et al. 2008). Thus, navigation systems in general seem to have a high accuracy. However, to achieve a high accuracy and avoid errors with navigation methods, the exact determination of anatomic landmarks is important. It was proven that some of the existing mechanical guides had a poor precision and accuracy (DiGioia et al. 1998), and surgeons have to be familiar with the use of this additional tool in order to avoid errors. Wassilew and colleagues conducted a prospective randomized controlled study of two groups of 40 patients each (Wassilew et al. 2012). They compared the results achieved using an ultrasound-based navigation system with the ones using an imageless navigation system with surface registration. They concluded that there was an improvement in cup positioning using ultrasound-based navigation compared to imageless navigation systems by reducing the outliers and achieving a higher accuracy of anteversion. In the first group, cup positioning was assisted by an ultrasound-based navigation system, and in the second group, the cup was assisted by an imageless navigation system with surface registration. However, these guides require an exact knowledge of patient orientation on the operating table. This is more complicated in patients in lateral decubitus position rather than in supine position. Furthermore, surgeons have to rely on their experience to modify the guides intraoperatively so as to avoid a malalignment of the cup. Especially in obese patients, the orientation for an adequate positioning of the acetabular cup is often very difficult and may lead to a suboptimal implant orientation. This may result in a wide discrepancy between the planned implant positioning and the final orientation (DiGioia III et al. 2002). Hasart et al. investigated the influence of body mass index (BMI) and the thickness of the soft tissue on the postoperative cup position and accuracy in the application of an ultrasound-based and a pointer-based navigation system (Hasart et al. 2010). According to their data, the accuracy of the ultrasound-based and pointer-based navigation systems is influenced by the BMI and the thickness of the soft tissue layer above the symphysis. However, ultrasound-based navigation seems to have certain advantages with thicker soft tissue layers, as seen in overweight and obese patients. The fact that obesity has a negative influence on the accuracy of imageless navigation was confirmed by Tsukada and

Wakui (Tsukada and Wakui 2010). They divided patients into obese (BMI ≥25) and nonobese (BMI <25) groups. The error in anteversion was significantly higher in the obese group (4.8°±2.5°) than in the nonobese group (3.2°±2.6°; p=0.01). Hohmann et al. investigated acetabular component position after THA in correlation to anteversion and inclination to anterior pelvic soft tissue thickness (Hohmann et al. 2011a). Thirty patients were operated on via an anterolateral approach in supine position using an imageless navigation system. The data did not reveal any significant relationships between BMI, soft tissue thickness, and final intraoperative or postoperative cup position. In addition, Fukui et al. also did not determine factors potentially affecting the accuracy of the intraoperative assessment, such as BMI and soft tissue thickness using the imageless navigation system OrthoPilot® (Fukui et al. 2010).

Critics of navigation systems in THA argue that the use of navigation systems is associated with additional costs, prolonged surgical time, and a learning curve for the usage of these devices, and point out that the cup can be positioned adequately without computer navigation.

The literature on the influence of navigation in THA on prolongation of surgery shows varying results. Thorey et al. found a prolongation of the operative time to be 4.8±3.8 min after the learning curve (Thorey et al. 2009). Similar results were presented by Kreuzer and Leffers (Kreuzer and Leffers 2011). They determined a mean surgical time for the navigation group of 56 min (range, 34–91 min) and 61 min (range, 33–119 min) for the nonnavigated group.

13.4 Conclusion

In conclusion, navigation tools (e.g., OrthoPilot®) provide surgeons with data on acetabular and femoral positioning such that leg length, femoral offset, and range of motion can be optimized in order to avoid malpositioning of the components and thereby reduce complication such as early joint dislocation, limited range of motion due to femoroacetabular impingement, and early implant wear due to edge loading and leg length discrepancies. However, surgeons have to be familiar with this tool and they should also be aware of the possible errors.

References

Aesculap (2012) Internet Communication. http://www.orthopilot.de/cps/rde/xchg/ae-orthopilot-de-int/hs.xsl/7321.html. Cited 17 June 2012

Beckmann J, Stengel D, Tingart M, Gotz J, Grifka J, Luring C (2009) Navigated cup implantation in hip arthroplasty. Acta Orthop 80:538–544

Clarke MT, Lee PT, Arora A, Villar RN (2003) Levels of metal ions after small- and large-diameter metal-on-metal hip arthroplasty. J Bone Joint Surg Br 85:913–917

Confalonieri N, Manzotti A, Montironi F, Pullen C (2008) Leg length discrepancy, dislocation rate, and offset in total hip replacement using a short modular stem: navigation vs conventional freehand. Orthopedics 31

Dastane M, Dorr LD, Tarwala R, Wan Z (2011) Hip offset in total hip arthroplasty: quantitative measurement with navigation. Clin Orthop Relat Res 469:429–436

DiGioia AM, Jaramaz B, Blackwell M, Simon DA, Morgan F, Moody JE, Nikou C, Colgan BD, Aston CA, Labarca RS, Kischell E, Kanade T (1998) The Otto Aufranc Award. Image guided navigation system to measure intraoperatively acetabular implant alignment. Clin Orthop Relat Res 355:8–22

DiGioia AM III, Jaramaz B, Plakseychuk AY, Moody JE Jr, Nikou C, Labarca RS, Levison TJ, Picard F (2002) Comparison of a mechanical acetabular alignment guide with computer placement of the socket. J Arthroplasty 17: 359–364

DiGioia AM, III, Plakseychuk AY, Levison TJ, Jaramaz B (2003) Mini-incision technique for total hip arthroplasty with navigation. J Arthroplasty 18:123–128

Dobzyniak M, Fehring TK, Odum S (2006) Early failure in total hip arthroplasty. Clin Orthop Relat Res 447:76–78

Fukui T, Fukunishi S, Nishio S, Shibanuma N, Yoshiya S (2010) Use of image-free navigation in determination of acetabular cup orientation: analysis of factors affecting precision. Orthopedics 33:38–42

Gebel P, Oszwald M, Ishaque B, Ahmed G, Blessing R, Thorey F, Ottersbach A (2012) Process optimized minimally invasive total hip replacement. Orthop Rev (Pavia) 4:e3

Gonzalez MH, Carr R, Walton S, Mihalko WM (2011) The Evolution and Modern Use of metal-on-metal bearings in total hip arthroplasty. Instr Course Lect 60:247–255

Hasart O, Perka C, Christian K, Asbach P, Janz V, Wassilew GI (2010) Influence of body mass index and thickness of soft tissue on accuracy of ultrasound and pointer based registration in navigation of cup in hip arthroplasty. Technol Health Care 18:341–351

Hohmann E, Bryant A, Tetsworth K (2011a) Anterior pelvic soft tissue thickness influences acetabular cup positioning with imageless navigation. J Arthroplasty 27:945–952

Hohmann E, Bryant A, Tetsworth K (2011b) Accuracy of acetabular cup positioning using imageless navigation. J Orthop Surg Res 6:40

Hohmann E, Bryant A, Tetsworth K (2011c) A comparison between imageless navigated and manual freehand technique acetabular cup placement in total hip arthroplasty. J Arthroplasty 26:1078–1082

Jacobs JJ, Hallab NJ, Skipor AK, Urban RM (2003) Metal degradation products: a cause for concern in metal-metal bearings? Clin Orthop Relat Res 139–147

Kennedy JG, Rogers WB, Soffe KE, Sullivan RJ, Griffen DG, Sheehan LJ (1998) Effect of acetabular component orientation on recurrent dislocation, pelvic osteolysis, polyethylene wear, and component migration. J Arthroplasty 13:530–534

Kreuzer S, Leffers K (2011) Direct anterior approach to total hip arthroplasty using computer navigation. Bull NYU Hosp Jt Dis 69 [Suppl 1]: S52–S55

Lewinnek GE, Lewis JL, Tarr R, Compere CL, Zimmerman JR (1978) Dislocations after total hip-replacement arthroplasties. J Bone Joint Surg Am 60:217–220

Lin F, Lim D, Wixson RL, Milos S, Hendrix RW, Makhsous M (2011) Limitations of imageless computer-assisted navigation for total hip arthroplasty. J Arthroplasty 26:596–605

McCollum DE, Gray WJ (1990) Dislocation after total hip arthroplasty. Causes and prevention. Clin Orthop Relat Res 159–170

Moskal JT, Capps SG (2011) Acetabular component positioning in total hip arthroplasty: an evidence-based analysis. J Arthroplasty 26:1432–1437

Nishikubo Y, Fujioka M, Ueshima K, Saito M, Kubo T (2011) Preoperative fluoroscopic imaging reduces variability of acetabular component positioning. J Arthroplasty 26:1088–1094

Nogler M (2004) Navigated minimal invasive total hip arthroplasty. Surg Technol Int 12:259–262

Nogler M, Mayr E, Krismer M, Thaler M (2008) Reduced variability in cup positioning: the direct anterior surgical approach using navigation. Acta Orthop 79:789–793

Parratte S, Argenson JN (2007) Validation and usefulness of a computer-assisted cup-positioning system in total hip arthroplasty. A prospective, randomized, controlled study. J Bone Joint Surg Am 89:494–499

Punwar S, Khan W S, Longo UG (2011) The use of computer navigation in hip arthroplasty: literature review and evidence today. Ortop Traumatol Rehabil 13:431–438

Renkawitz T, Tingart M, Grifka J, Sendtner E, Kalteis T (2009) Computer-assisted total hip arthroplasty: coding the next generation of navigation systems for orthopedic surgery. Expert Rev Med Devices 6:507–514

Schmalzried TP, Guttmann D, Grecula M, Amstutz HC (1994) The relationship between the design, position, and articular wear of acetabular components inserted without cement and the development of pelvic osteolysis. J Bone Joint Surg Am 76:677–688

Sendtner E, Muller M, Winkler R, Worner M, Grifka J, Renkawitz T (2010) Femur first in hip arthroplasty--the concept of combined anteversion (in German). Z Orthop Unfall 148:185–190

Snyder GM, Calderon SA, Lucas PA, Russinoff S (2012) Accuracy of computer-navigated total hip arthroplasty. J Arthroplasty 27:415–420

Sotereanos NG, Miller MC, Smith B, Hube R, Sewecke JJ, Wohlrab D (2006) Using intraoperative pelvic landmarks for acetabular component placement in total hip arthroplasty. J Arthroplasty 21:832–840

Thorey F, Klages P, Lerch M, Florkemeier T, Windhagen H, von Lewinski G (2009) Cup positioning in primary total hip arthroplasty using an imageless navigation device: is there a learning curve? Orthopedics 32:14–17

Tsukada S, Wakui M (2010) Decreased accuracy of acetabular cup placement for imageless navigation in obese patients. J Orthop Sci 15:758–763

Turner RS (1994) Postoperative total hip prosthetic femoral head dislocations. Incidence, etiologic factors, and management. Clin Orthop Relat Res 301:196–204

Vendittoli PA, Roy A, Mottard S, Girard J, Lusignan D, Lavigne M (2010) Metal ion release from bearing wear and corrosion with 28 mm and large-diameter metal-on-metal bearing articulations: a follow-up study. J Bone Joint Surg Br 92:12–19

Wassilew GI, Perka C, Janz V, Konig C, Asbach P, Hasart O (2012) Use of an ultrasound-based navigation system for an accurate acetabular positioning in total hip arthroplasty: a prospective, randomized, controlled study. J Arthroplasty 27:687–694

Widmer KH, Zurfluh B (2004) Compliant positioning of total hip components for optimal range of motion. J Orthop Res 22:815–821

Williamson JA, Reckling FW (1978) Limb length discrepancy and related problems following total hip joint replacement. Clin Orthop Relat Res 134:135–138

Yuan L, Shih C (1999) Dislocation after total hip arthroplasty. Arch Orthop Trauma Surg 119:263–266

Short Stem Navigation and Optimized Range of Motion

Djordje Lazovic

The demand for less invasive procedures and bone-sparing hip implants has led to the development of short stem prostheses. Various types of hip prostheses are called short stem, although they are based on different principles. Shortened conventional, short anatomic, double taper type, and neck implants rely on different fixation points in the femur and need to be reviewed individually. Short stem prostheses all have in common that they preserve the greater trochanter and part of the femoral neck, which leads to a curved implantation technique and is well suited for a minimally invasive procedure. The cementless fixed prostheses provide a high primary stability to allow immediate weight bearing (Eingartner 2007).

14.1 Introduction

The implant used in our series has a double taper design as first introduced by Morrey (Morrey 1989). It relies on a multipoint fixation with cortical contact at the medial calcar, the lateral rim of the resected neck, as well as the distal appendix in the posterior lateral subtrochanteric region. Unfortunately, because these implants are designed to follow the anatomical shape of the femoral neck they do not have an influence on the final orientation (Morrey et al. 2000). This final position determines the position of the implants in the femoral neck, probably changing offset and leg length as well as the center of rotation. Müller et al. (2011) and Sendtner et al. (2010) described the effect of implant tilt and implant rotation on the reconstruction of the center of rotation in hip reconstruction, respectively.

In slim straight stem designs, the implant can be rotated in the femoral canal to adjust for pathologic ante- or retroversion. The different fixation in »femoral neck-preserving designs« does not allow for this correction. For this to be achieved, a separation of femoral fixation and a reconstruction of the biomechanics are desirable. This can be achieved by modularity. In the modular implant used in these cases, three different caput collum diaphysis (CCD) angles of the neck module can be used (130°, 135°, and 140°) each with a retroverted, neutral, and anteverted orientation (−7.5°/0°/+7.5°) to adjust the offset, leg length, and center of rotation (Braun 2007, 2009, Lazovic 2006, Milecki et al. 2008).

Correct adjustment is a matter of discussion (D'Lima et al. 2000, 2001; Dorr 2009; Matsuhita et al. 2010; Renkawitz et al. 2011; Seki et al. 1998). Most authors prefer an anatomic reconstruction, but the concept of a combined anteversion is receiving increasing attention. In our series we emphasize the importance of a high range of motion (ROM) without impingement.

The choice of the best geometry for achieving this goal has to take into account the center of rotation, the changes of offset, leg length, and the version of the femoral neck, in this case of the modular connector between the short stem implant and the femoral head. To find the optimum, a trial-and-error method with different sample connectors and head length has the disadvantage of taking time and requiring multiple reductions and dislocations of the hip. We can simulate these trials on the screen of our routinely used navigation system (Fig. 14.1). The screen offers information on the version of the stem in relation to the femur, the leg extension, and the offset changes and it displays the ROM in flexion, in external rotation for the extended leg, and in internal rotation for the 90° flexed leg. The parameters can be changed on the screen to evaluate the effect on the ROM values. The changes account for the CCD angle (125°, 130°, 135°, and 140°), the version (−7.5°, 0°, *7.5°), and the head length (S, M, L, XL) and head size (28 mm, 32 mm, 36 mm). All of these values can be individually adjusted and the effect on ROM can be seen immediately (Fig. 14.2). The ideal setting is then chosen. According to our experience, minimum values of 110° flexion, 30° internal rotation, and 60° external rotation are accepted and assessed as safe for the lateral or anterolateral approach. For the posterior and direct anterior approach, values may differ.

14.2 Surgical Technique for Short Stem Prostheses

In our series, all short stem prostheses were implanted via a minimized anterolateral Watson–Jones approach, bluntly separating the gluteus medius and the lateral vastus muscle. The capsule is opened in a »door type« manner and closed if appropriate. In tight soft tissue situations, a soft tissue release is per-

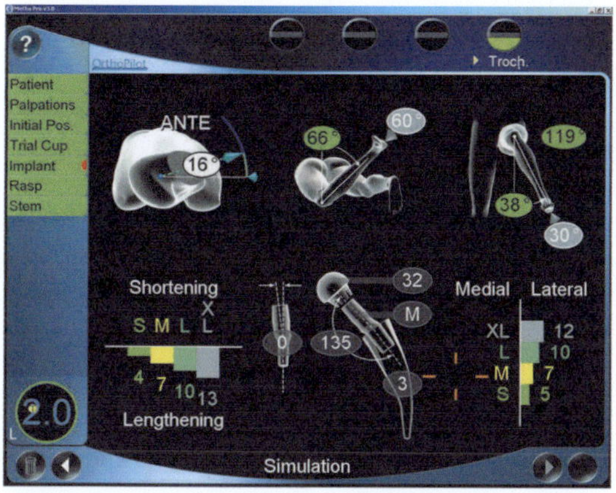

Fig. 14.1 The simulation screen allows one to change the values of the CCD angle as well as the ante- or retrotorsion; it displays the changes in the values for antetorsion of the femoral neck and the range of motion. (By courtesy of B. Braun, Aesculap)

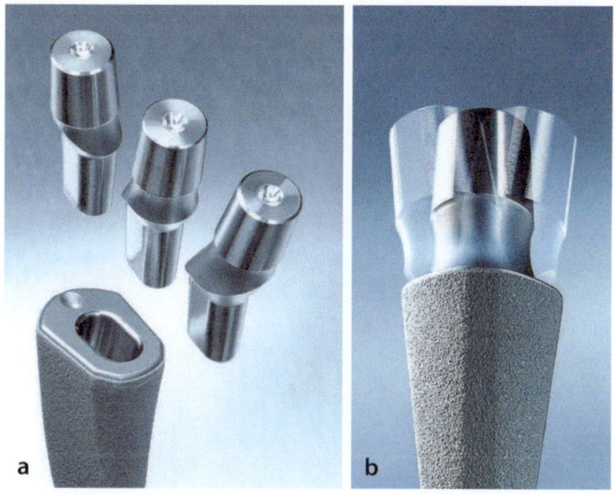

Fig. 14.2 The modular connector allows for adjustment of the CCD angle (**a**) and the ante-/retrotorsion (**b**). (By courtesy of B. Braun, Aesculap)

formed and the capsule is resected. The femoral neck is cut after dislocation of the femoral head about 5 mm medial to the greater trochanter in a 50° angle.

The cup is prepared first. We routinely started at a position of 45° inclination and 15° anteversion of the cup. In our series, the majority of patients had dysplastic hip arthritis with the wellknown deformities of a poor anterior coverage of the acetabulum and an increased antetorsion of the femoral neck up to 50°. In these cases we plan the cup position in a reduced anteversion of 10°. All cups are hemispherical, cementless, fixed, and in a few cases secured by an additional screw. The insert is ceramic.

The femoral intramedullary canal is opened with an awl and then rasped until a tight fit in the femoral neck is achieved. Usually, the edges of the nearly rectangular-shaped prosthesis reach the cortical contact on the calcar and the lateral flange reaches the cortical border of the proximal femoral neck. This places the prosthesis in a direction mainly defined by the direction of the natural femoral neck. After choosing and inserting the best fitting femoral neck and head, the hip is reduced, dislocation tests are performed, and x-rays taken to verify the stem and cup position and to check the integrity of the pelvis and femur. The capsule and wound are then closed. Immediate weight bearing is allowed 1 day after surgery. Limitations are given for the first 6 weeks for flexion up to 90°, avoiding adduction and external rotation.

14.3 Navigation Technique

Before approaching the hip, a rigid body is fixed to the pelvis, about 5 cm lateral to the anterior superior iliac spine via an 8-mm incision. The anterior pelvic plane is recorded by palpating the anterior ipsilateral and contralateral iliac spines and the symphysis using a pointer. After access to the femur, a rigid body is fixed using a C-clamp and the neutral leg position is recorded. The axis of the femur is determined by palpation of the center of the patella in the 90° flexed knee. The version of the femoral neck is calculated by recording the posterior condyles pointing at the middle of the ankle in the 90° flexed knee. After resection of the femoral head, the depth and the natural anatomic version of the acetabulum are recorded.

Reaming of the acetabulum is controlled by navigation, giving information on depth, version, and changes of the center in anterior/posterior, medial/lateral, and proximal/distal direction. The hemispherical cup is inserted using the previously recorded information specifically aiming for values of 45° inclination and 10° anteversion.

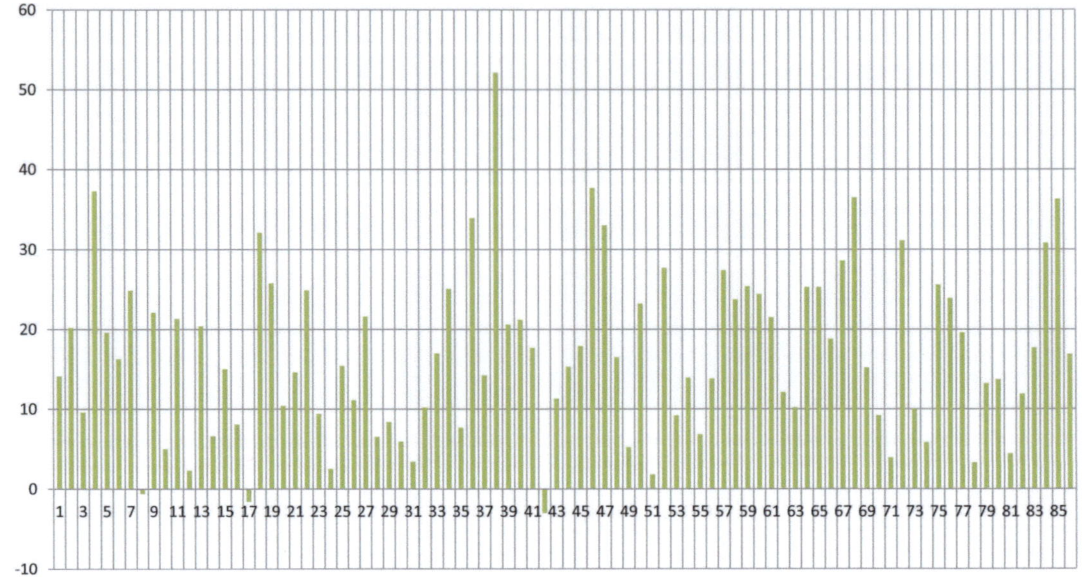

Fig. 14.3 Postoperative antetorsion values of the femoral neck, corrected with modular connectors; mean, 16.9°

After reaming and inserting the stem, which is done by focusing entirely on the best fitting position, the implant position is recorded by the navigation system. Based on these values, the simulation screen allows a decision to be made on the best fitting modular connector and head.

A final screen shows the changes in offset and leg length by bringing the leg back into its original neutral position.

14

14.4 Results

From November 2004 to December 2010 we implanted 322 short stem prostheses (Metha®, B. Braun) in the manner described above. In 297 cases the cup and stem were navigated, while in 65 cases the stem was implanted without navigation. Of our patients 176 were female and 146 were male; the mean body mass index (BMI) was 27.1. The etiology of coxarthritis was primary osteoarthritis in 144 cases, dysplasia in 109, femoral head necrosis in 35, and secondary coxarthritis in 34 cases. The mean cup size was 52 mm in diameter with a range of 44–66 mm, the mean stem size was 3 with a range of 0–7. We used 119 modular connectors with a CCD angle of 130°, 148 with 135°, and 55 with 140°. In 17 cases we increased the antetorsion of the femoral neck with +7.5° anteverted connector, in 139 the antetorsion remained unchanged with a neutral 0° connector, and in 166 the antetorsion was decreased with a −7.5° connector.

With these adjustments we achieved a mean ROM of 130.9° of flexion, 70.3° of external rotation in straight leg position, and 50.7° of internal rotation in a 90° flexed position of the hip.

It was not possible to achieve the optimum position in every case. Owing to fixation difficulties, cup inclination varied from 39° to 58° with a mean of 45.2°, and anteversion varied from 0° to 41° with a mean of 15.2°. The stem antetorsion varied according to the natural variability from −5.3° to 56.6° with a mean of 20.6°. The ROM for internal and external rotation correlated with the values of the cup position for anteversion and for combined anteversion.

Combined anteversion, adding the values of stem antetorsion and cup anteversion, was 36.3° (variation of 2.2°–82.2°). Clinical results showed no dislocations.

The effect of modular connectors on the correction of decreased or increased femoral neck antetorsion was checked for the last 86 implants. The original, noncorrected antetorsion was calculated from the registered data in the navigation

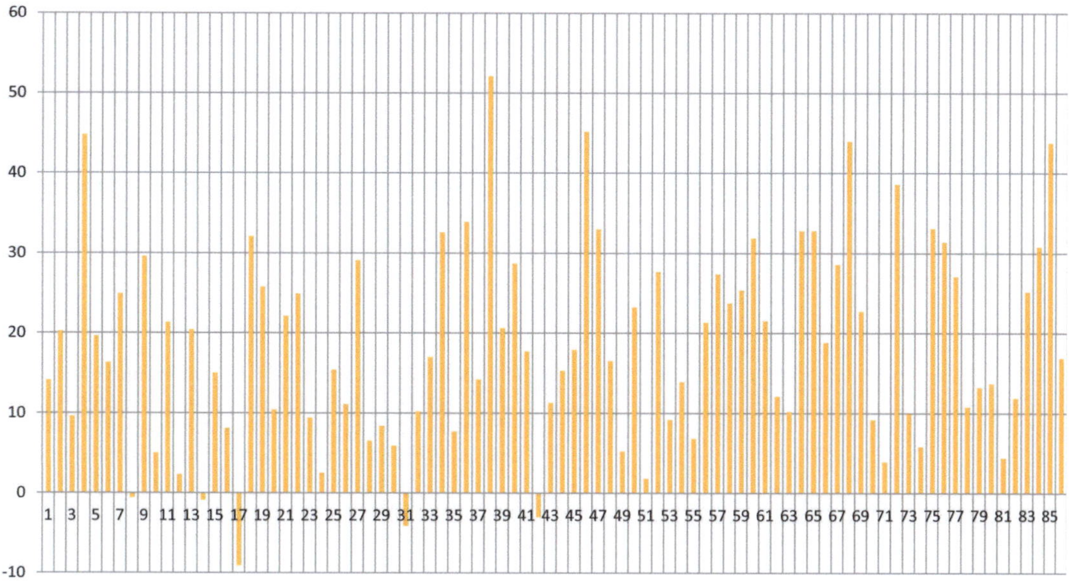

Fig. 14.4 Calculated antetorsion of the femoral neck if no correction would have been used; mean, 18.4°

computer. The mean antetorsion was 18.4° for the natural femoral neck and 16.9° for the corrected modular connectors (Fig. 14.3, Fig. 14.4). The correction was not sufficient to bring the values into the nonpathological area of 10°–25°. The highest values corrected were +52° and –2°.

14.5 Discussion

The effect of implant position on geometry and biomechanics in hip reconstruction and their influence on function is intensively discussed.

Lewinnek (Lewinnek et al. 1978) investigated the best position for cup placement to avoid dislocation in respect to anteversion and inclination. These values are still recommended for THA and known as the »Lewinnek safe zone.« A reduction in the incidence of dislocations can be achieved when the cup is placed in this zone. Navigation of the cup aims at this goal of an ideal cup position and reduces the outliers significantly.

However, dislocations still occur, and with a wider use of THA in younger patients expectations for a better function and increased ROM grow. It is obvious that hip function is influenced by both the cup and the stem. Restoring leg length and offset results in a better muscular function. This is also emphasized by minimally invasive surgical techniques using short stems.

Straight or anatomically shaped cementless femoral stems have only a limited variability regarding their position in the femur (Renkawitz et al. 2012). In short stems the fixation in the metaphysis allows for nearly no changes of the anatomic preconditions. This position determines the center of rotation of the femoral head. When an optimum of safe, dislocation- and impingement-free ROM is addressed, the surgeon has to take into account leg length, offset, center of rotation, femoral stem antetorsion and tilt, as well as head neck ratio and their relation to the cup position with respect to inclination and anteversion (Fig. 14.5).

Combined antetorsion of the cup and stem is viewed as an aid in finding this optimum (Sariali 2009a, 2009b). Published values show a mean combined antetorsion of 37.6° (Dorr 2009) and 34.4° (Wassilew 2012). In our series it is 36.3°. The safe range is claimed to be 25°–50° (Dorr 2009), but this depends on the surgical approach. The variation in our series is much higher than that is reported in the literature. The reason might be the use of a short stem that allows an adjustment of the anatomically preconditioned antetorsion to be made only by a

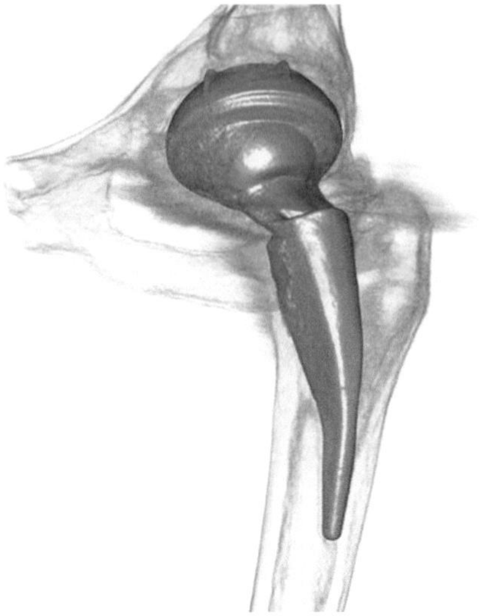

Fig. 14.5 A three-dimensional computed tomography scan shows the fit and fill placement of the short stem in the femoral metaphysis, determining the orientation of the femoral neck and the relation to the acetabular cup

modular neck. This modular connector has a limited correction value of ±7.5°, which is not enough to reach a mean antetorsion of the femoral stem of 15°, which should be the ideal value. The high number of dysplastic hips with an antetorsion deformity in our series resulted in a mean antetorsion of 16.9° even with modular correction and 18.4° without correction. Consequently, we decided to reduce the cup anteversion from 15°, as demanded by Lewinnek, to 10° in all dysplastic cases.

The modularity helps to adjust the offset and leg length by different CCD angles. To find the optimum, connector navigation is an important tool. The simulation screen displays the values for the ROM depending on the adjustments made first on the screen for CCD and head size and length, and it allows the combined antetorsion to be calculated. Subsequently, the neck that best fits the desired ROM is chosen and assembled to the stem. The high mean ROM in flexion and in internal and external rotation has resulted in clinically stable hips without dislocation as seen at follow-up in our series.

References

Braun A, Sabah A (2009) Two-year results of a modular short hip stem prosthesis – a prospective study. Z Orthop Unfall 147:700–706

Braun A, Lazovic D, Zigan R (2007) Modular short-stem prosthesis in total hip arthroplasty: implant positioning and the influence of navigation. Orthopedics 30:S148–152

D'Lima DD, Urquhart AG, Buehler KO, Walker RH, Colwell CW Jr (2000) The effect of the orientation of the acetabular and femoral components on the range of motion of the hip at different head-neck ratios. J Bone Joint Surg Am 82:315–321

D'Lima DD, Chen PC, Colwell CW Jr (2001) Optimizing acetabular component position to minimize impingement and reduce contact stress. J Bone Joint Surg Am 83:87–91

Dorr LD, Malik A, Dastane M, Wan Z (2009) Combined anteversion technique for total hip arthroplasty. Clin Orthop Relat Res 467:119–127

Eingartner C (2007) Currents trends in total hip arthroplasty. Orthop Traumatol Rehabil 9:8–14

Lazovic D, Zigan R (2006/7) Navigation of short-stem implants. Orthopedics 29:S125–129. Erratum in: Orthopedics 30:327

Lewinnek GE, Lewis JL, Tarr R, Compere CL, Zimmerman JR (1978) Dislocations after total hip replacement arthroplasties. J Bone Joint Surg Am 60:217–220

Matsushita A, Nakashima Y, Fujii M, Sato T, Iwamoto Y (2010) Modular necks improve the range of hip motion in cases with excessively anteverted or retroverted femurs in THA. Clin Orthop Relat Res 468:3342–3347

Milecki M, Kowalczewski J, Wielopolski A, Obrebski M, Okoń T, Marczak D (2008) Modular short-stem prosthesis in total hip arthroplasty – preliminary report (in Polish). Chir Narzadow Ruchu Ortop Pol 73:244–247

Morrey BF (1989) Short-stemmed uncemented femoral component for primary hip arthroplasty. Clin Orthop Relat Res 249:169–175

Morrey BF, Adams RA, Kessler M (2000) A conservative femoral replacement for total hip arthroplasty. A prospective study. J Bone Joint Surg Br 82:952–958

Müller M, Crucius D, Perka C, Tohtz S (2011) The association between the sagittal femoral stem alignment and the resulting femoral head centre in total hip arthroplasty. Int Orthop (SICOT) 35:981–987

Renkawitz T, Haimerl M, Dohmen L, Gneiting S, Wegner M, Ehret N, Buchele C, Schubert M, Lechler P, Woerner M, Sendtner E, Schuster T, Ulm K, Springorum R, Grifka J (2011) Minimally invasive computer-navigated total hip arthroplasty, following the concept of femur first and combined anteversion: design of a blinded randomized controlled trial. BMC Musculoskelet Disord 12:192

Renkawitz T, Haimerl M, Dohmen L, Gneiting S, Lechler P, Woerner M, Springorum HR, Weber M, Sussmann P, Sendtner E, Grifka J (2012) The association between femoral tilt and impingement-free range-of-motion in total hip arthroplasty. BMC Musculoskelet Disord 13:65

Sariali E, Mouttet A, Pasquier G, Durante E (2009a) Three-dimensional hip anatomy in osteoarthritis. Analysis of the femoral offset. J Arthroplasty 24:990–997

Sariali E, Mouttet A, Pasquier G, Durante E, Catone Y (2009b) Accuracy of reconstruction of the hip using computerised three-dimensional pre-operative planning and a cementless modular neck. J Bone Joint Surg Br 91:333–340

Seki M, Yuasa N, Ohkuni K (1998) Analysis of optimal range of socket orientations in total hip arthroplasty with use of computer-aided design simulation. J Orthop Res 16:513–517

Sendtner E, Tibor S, Winkler R, Wörner M, Grifka J, Renkawitz T (2010) Stem torsion in total hip replacement. Acta Orthop 81:579–582

Wassilew GI, Perka C, Koenig C, Janz V, Asbach P, Hasart O (2012) 3D CT analysis of combined cup and stem anteversion in cases of cup navigation in hip arthroplasty. Orthopedics 33:48–51

Ultrasound-Guided Acquisition of Bony Landmarks During Navigation

Hartmuth Kiefer

In navigated implantation of an artificial hip replacement, the surgeon receives data for aligning the acetabulum and prosthetic stem and matching the cup and stem position to one another during surgery. Prerequisite to this is reliable registration of bony landmarks in order to judge the anatomic and patient-specific situation. With image-assisted navigation systems, this can be accomplished by means of surface matching on the basis of preoperative computed tomography (CT) data or percutaneous registration under fluoroscopic control.
With kinematic, imageless navigation systems, navigated pointers are used to obtain intraoperative point registrations of acetabular and femoral landmarks. During direct registrations, bony landmarks on the acetabulum or femur can be taken directly in situ at the bone surface. During indirect registrations as in the anterior pelvic plane, there is a soft tissue cover that distorts the registration result.

15.1 Introduction

During hip navigation, the anterior pelvic plane (APP) is the reference plane for establishing the inclination and anteversion angle of the cup. Registration is accomplished by using a pointer to palpate both the anterior superior iliac spine (ASIS) and the symphysis. The soft tissue covering the symphysis can lead to false interpretation of the anteversion by 8.2° (min. 2°, max. 24°) on average. The value is displayed as if the anteversion value were higher (Richolt and Rittmeister 2006).

Spencer et al. recruited eight surgeons to investigate the influence of various percutaneous palpation points of the anterior pelvic plane on human cadavers. At a standard deviation of 9.6°, the variation in anteversion was higher than for the inclination, which had a standard deviation of 6.3° (Spencer et al. 2006). Lee and Yoon determined the palpation errors of a kinematic navigation system at registration deviations of 10 mm on the landmarks of the pelvic entrance plane using a pelvic model and found higher deviations for the acetabulum anteversion and only minimal deviations for the inclination (Lee and Yoon 2008).

The use of ultrasound to visualize bony tissue was described by Tretbar and colleagues (Tretbar et al. 2002). Attempts at ultrasound registration of bone lengths, axes, and torsion positions (Keppler et al. 2007) showed high precision in the range of 1 mm and 1° of angle. Parratte and colleagues confirmed the high measurement accuracy of 1 mm with a hand-guided ultrasound transducer during registration of the anterior pelvic plane on human cadavers (Parratte et al. 2008). By comparing ultrasound and pointer registration in the clinical implementation of a hip navigation system, Hirschmann et al. reported deviations in the median acetabulum anteversion of 6° (range, 3°–13°) and in the median inclination of 3° (range, −1°–5°) for ultrasound registration as compared to pointer registration (Hirschmann et al. 2011).

Ultrasound registration with the navigation system OrthoPilot® (B. Braun, Aesculap AG, Tuttlingen, Germany) has been available in our clinic since 2006. In a pilot study with 37 consecutive navigated total hip replacements implanted by navigation, we compared percutaneous pointer registration with ultrasound registration, showing an approximately fivefold improvement in the anteversion registration accuracy with regards to the radiological cup position on the postoperative radiographs. Especially in overweight patients, pointer palpation of the symphysis can cause difficulty because of the large amounts of soft and fatty tissue in the area to be palpated. Particularly in such cases, the postoperative radiographs will often show a lower cup anteversion compared to the values determined intraoperatively by palpation. The registration of symphysis landmarks by ultrasound is not affected by overlying fatty tissue (◘ Fig. 15.1, ◘ Tab. 15.1) (Kiefer and Othman 2007).

Comparison of cup anteversion measurements showed significantly higher values for ultrasound registration as compared to pointer registration (p=0.000001). In turn, pointer registration produced significantly higher anteversion values than postoperative radiographs (p=0.0001).

In two groups of 30 patients each matched by gender, age, body mass index (BMI), and ASA (American Society of Anesthesiologists classification) for ultrasound and pointer registration, navigated THA procedures employing the same navigation system showed a significant improvement in anteversion deviation as compared to percutaneous

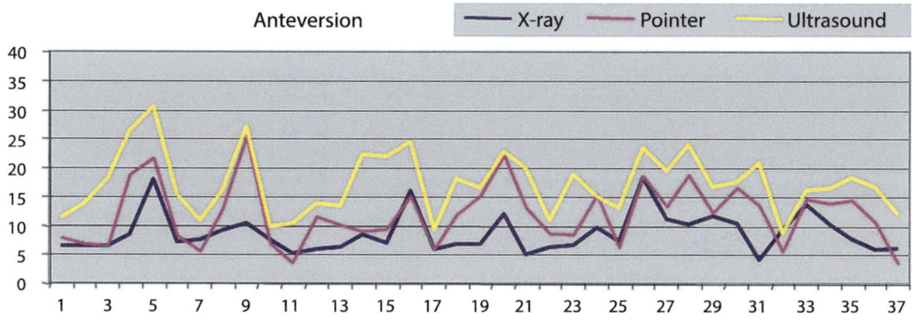

Fig. 15.1 Comparative analysis of the acetabulum anteversion angle on postoperative radiographs in 37 cases based on data from intraoperative pointer registrations and intraoperative ultrasound registrations. (Kiefer and Othman 2007)

Tab. 15.1 Deviations in anteversion values (Kiefer and Othman 2007)

	Average	SD
Anteversion radiograph	11.9	5.3
Pointer without radiograph	3.2	4.2
Ultrasound without radiograph	8.7	4.5
Ultrasound without pointer	5.5	3.3

pointer registration; the improvements in inclination were not significant (Hasart et al. 2008). CT follow-up studies of ultrasound-navigated acetabular cup positioning in 25 patients showed equal deviations of 2.8° (SD±1.8°) for inclination and 2.2° (SD±1.6°) for anteversion (Hasart et al. 2009).

In a prospective, randomized two-group study (Wassilew et al. 2012) on 80 patients, three-dimensional postoperative CT scans were used to determine cup position accuracy obtained with ultrasound navigation as compared to that obtained with imageless navigation by percutaneous pointer palpation.

All patients were operated on in the supine position using a minimally invasive anterolateral approach. Based on postoperative CT scans, a three-dimensional pelvic model was visualized with modeling software to achieve accurate determination of the implant position in each patient. The aim of the three-dimensional visualization of the implant position was to rule out the influence of postoperative pelvic tilt on accurate acetabular cup position. The objective for the position of the acetabular implant component was the Lewinnek »safe zone,« with an inclination of 40° and an anteversion of 15°.

The study results showed a significant difference in anteversion when comparing ultrasound-based navigation to imageless navigation (p=0.0001). Furthermore, in the group with imageless navigation, 12 of 40 (30%) acetabular components were implanted outside of the Lewinnek safe zone, while only one case (2.5%) was outside of the Lewinnek safe zone in the group using ultrasound-based navigation. Additionally, in the group with imageless navigation, a significant dependence was identified between the anteversion values and BMI. However, no such significance was observed in the group with ultrasound-based navigation. Therefore, the accuracy of imageless navigation with percutaneous palpation is negatively influenced by the patient's BMI, while ultrasound-based palpation improves the accuracy of anterior pelvic plane registration.

15.2 The Technology Behind Ultrasound Navigation

OrthoPilot® ultrasound navigation relies on linear array-based, two-dimensional ultrasound imaging technology. A transducer with a width of 80 mm has proven effective to sufficiently visualize the pelvic anatomy. For the visualization of bony tissue, the system produces ultrasound signals at a frequency of 3–7 MHz by means of 128-element piezoelectric, pulse-echo technology. It is thus possible to identify bony structures at a depth of up to 80 mm with a maximum deviation of 1.7 mm per axis during registration of the anterior pelvic plane.

The ultrasound transducer is used in a sterile operating environment. As the transducer is non-autoclavable, a sterile barrier is created using a sterile sleeve. This sterile barrier, by definition, is perforated when fixating the adapter for the navigation transducer. Therefore, a special validated interface for fixating the navigation transducer was developed; its microbial impermeability has been verified by an independent institute.

The OrthoPilot® ultrasound application is equipped with a specific ultrasound parameter set for navigation during total hip arthroplasty. The surgeon, therefore, does not have to set any parameters such as focal points, gain, or contrast that impact ultrasound imaging. Additionally, the characteristic feature of navigated ultrasound devices is that the ultrasound transducer can identify the position of the ultrasound plane within a fixed coordinate system. The position of each ultrasound plane is specific to the individual transducer. That is why the ultrasound transducer is integrated once into the navigation software by means of a single calibration and then permanently saved in an EPROM module. This is unique for the OrthoPilot® system, as all navigable instruments are otherwise produced and designed uniformly so they can be used with different OrthoPilot® navigation systems without single calibration.

The exact ultrasound imaging procedure and proper guidance of the ultrasound transducer are presented in Sect. 15.4 on »Ultrasound Visualization and Transducer Guidance.«

15.3 Intraoperative Prerequisites

During the preparations for surgery, the ultrasound transducer is sterilized by means of a sterile sleeve. As described above, the adapter for the infrared receiver (Rigid Body Adapter) is connected to the transducer through the sleeve. The transducer is placed on the patient's skin after using a sterile ultrasound gel, which is applied in small amounts to the transducer or the part of the patient's body being scanned using a 10 ml syringe. The areas to be palpated can be taped off with a sterile incision drape, taking care to avoid air bubbles, as they interfere with ultrasound transduction (Fig. 15.2, Fig. 15.3, Fig. 15.4).

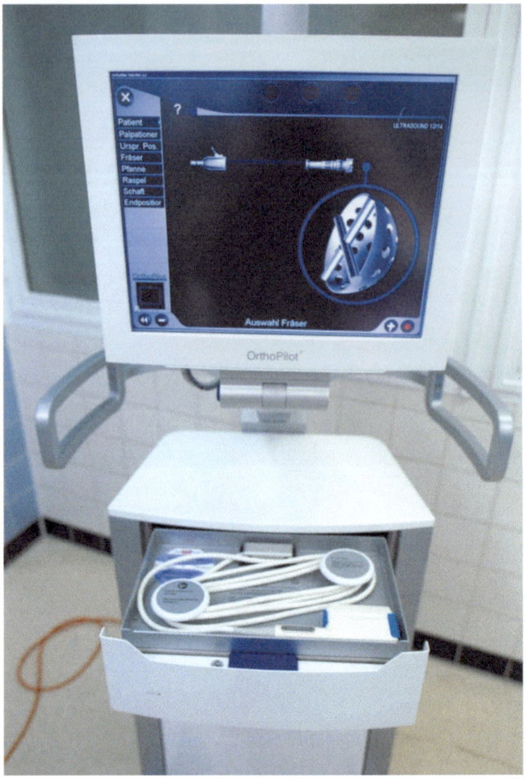

Fig. 15.2 OrthoPilot® Navigation system (B. Braun, Aesculap AG, Tuttlingen) with ultrasound unit

15.4 Ultrasound Visualization and Transducer Guidance

The image captured by the ultrasound transducer represents a two-dimensional sectional plane, in which the bony surface contours are displayed as a line. For optimal visualization and alignment of the bony palpation planes, the surgeon guides and places the ultrasound transducer vertical to the bone surface and along the anatomic orientation of the landmarks to be palpated. This means that, to visualize the anterior superior iliac spine, the ultrasound transducer must also capture the anterior inferior iliac spine (Fig. 15.5, Fig15.6).

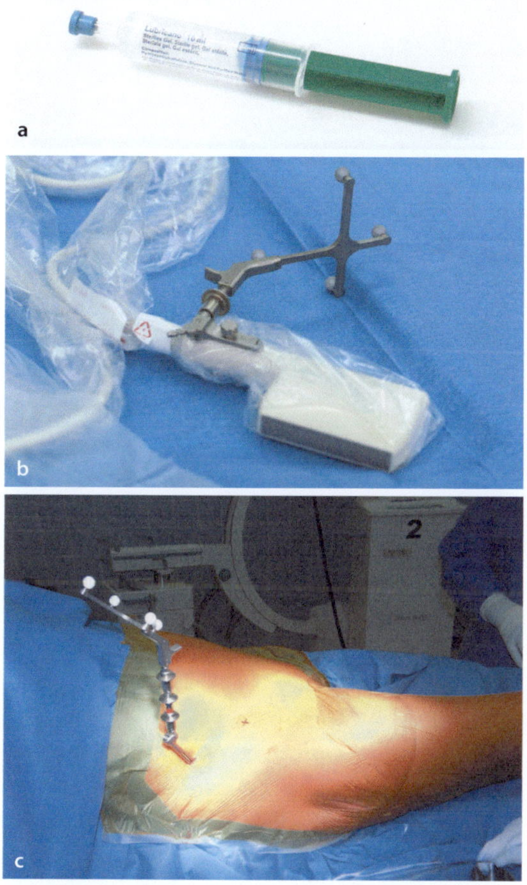

Fig. 15.3a–c Ultrasound navigation. **a** Sterile ultrasound gel (10 ml syringe). **b** An 80-mm ultrasound transducer with navigation transducer (Rigid Body). **c** Draping the patient for anterior pelvic plane registration during hip navigation

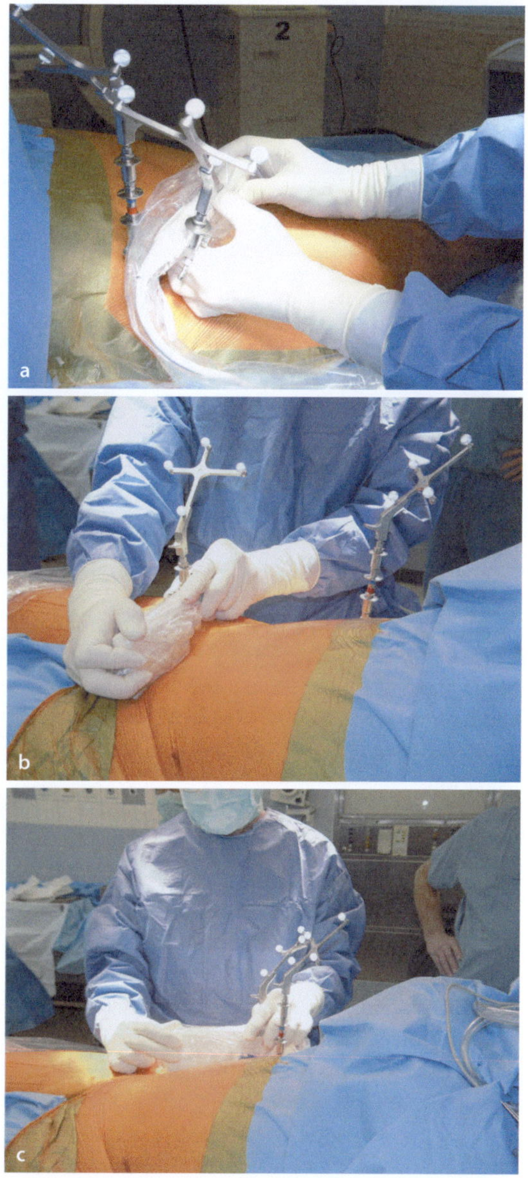

Fig. 15.4a–c Ultrasound registration of the anterior pelvic plane during hip navigation. Anterior superior iliac spine (ASIS) ipsilateral (**a**), ASIS contralateral (**b**), and symphysis (**c**)

The superior iliac spine must be selected as a landmark with a virtual pointer. This must take place ipsilaterally and contralaterally according to the same anatomical criteria. To visualize the two pubic tubercles, the ultrasound transducer is guided vertically to the anterior pelvic plane. The registration point is placed centrally over the symphysis, on a line connecting the tubercles.

In order to take advantage of the high accuracy of ultrasound registration, the registration can also be »guided«. During a test registration, the navigation system displays the anterior pelvic plane as a line on the ultrasound that can be corrected by a second registration.

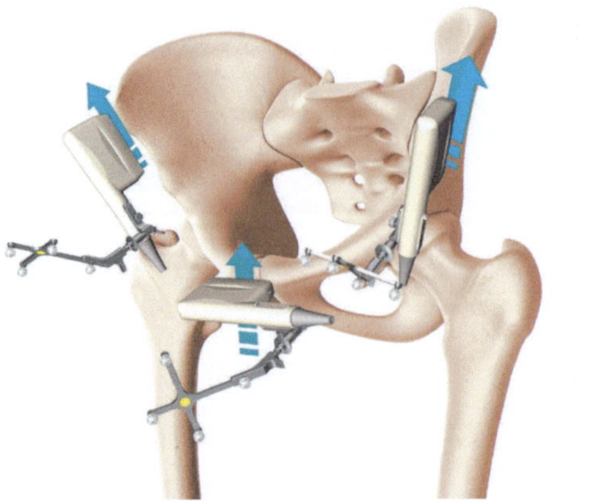

Fig. 15.5 Aligning and guiding the ultrasound transducer for registration of the anterior pelvic plane

15.5 Ultrasound Navigation in Total Hip Arthroplasty

Registration of landmarks to visualize the anterior pelvic plane (APP) by ultrasound generally offers a higher level of accuracy during navigation than visualization of the APP using percutaneous pointer palpation.

Navigated implantation of the acetabular components is the most commonly used technique for this, and can be combined with additional parameters for stem implantation. In order for the navigation system to recognize the position of the pelvis, the stabile fixation of a reference transducer on the anterior superior iliac spine is necessary for the entire duration of the navigation. This is accomplished on the ipsilateral side of the hip through an approximately 1 cm long puncture incision made around 5 cm posterior to the ipsilateral anterior superior iliac spine; an adapter is fixed with a special fixation screw and the pelvic reference transducer is adapted. The transducer should be aligned facing in the camera position.

After referencing the anterior pelvic plane by ultrasound, the position of the acetabulum is also referenced. Initial referencing takes place using a navigated trial cup, which helps the surgeon determine the anatomical situation. This provides the navigation system with an initial measurement for the hip joint center, while displaying the inclination and anteversion position of the trial cup. For these values, it must be taken into consideration that the subimplant bed has not yet been reamed at this point in time (Fig15.6).

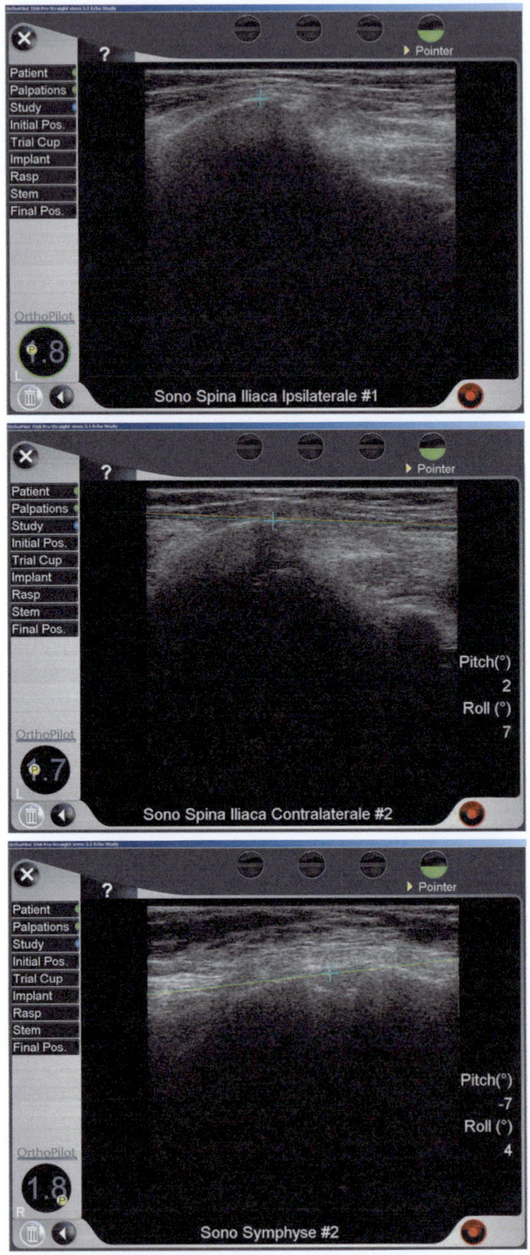

a

b

c

Fig15.6a–c Sonographic visualization for ultrasound registration of the anterior pelvic plane during hip navigation. ASIS ipsilateral (**a**), ASIS contralateral (**b**), and symphysis (c)

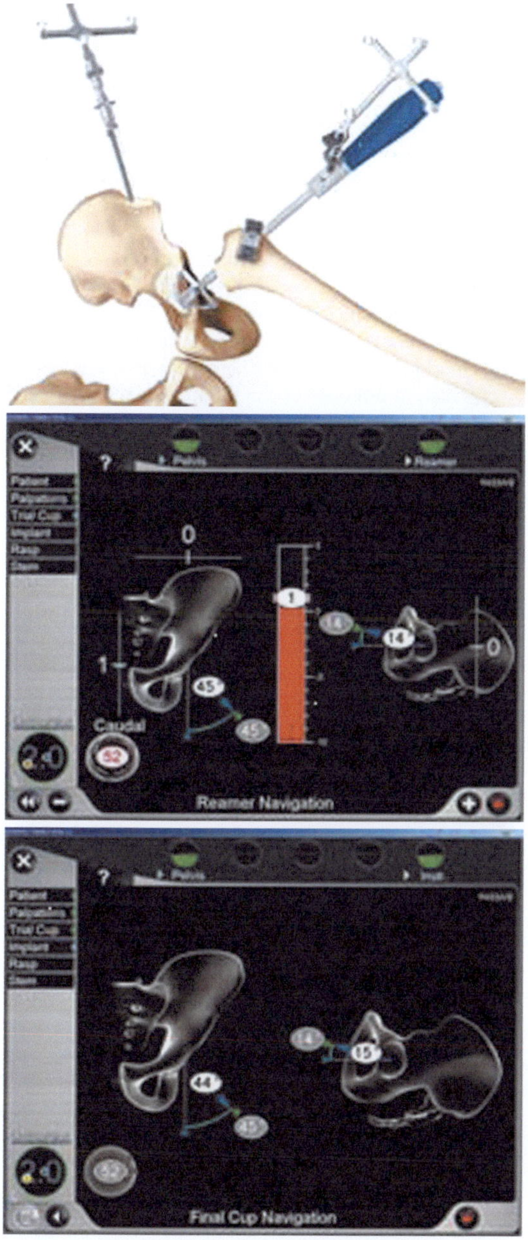

a b c

■ **Fig. 15.7a–c Procedural steps for acetabular cup navigation. a** Insert a navigated trial cup to determine the joint center and verify the anatomical alignment of the acetabulum. **b** Perform navigated reaming of the acetabulum. **c** Insert acetabular components under navigation

It is additionally possible to palpate bony points in the acetabulum, e.g., the deepest site within the acetabular fossa, using a pointer (in order to display or demarcate the reaming depth) or points on the acetabular rim; this supplies the navigation system with patient-matched information on acetabular anatomy.

Next, the surgeon can start preparing the acetabulum by navigated reaming. The angles for inclination and anteversion relative to the pelvic entrance plane are displayed on the screen. During this surgical step, these angles are helpful for determining the direction of reaming and verifying the navigation data. In the example shown here of the monitor, the surgeon is provided with additional data (in millimeters) on the reaming depth (red scale) as well as on the three-dimensional displacement of the hip center in the cranial, medial, and anterior/posterior directions. Two values on a gray background on the monitor indicate the initial acetabular inclination and anteversion as registered with the trial cup. The newly calculated acetabular center can thus be prepared according to the preoperative plan (■ Fig. 15.7).

Just as with conventional operative techniques, secure anchoring of the cup implant is the primary goal of navigation assisted surgery. Therefore, the acetabular cup's system-specific characteristics must be taken into consideration when preparing the implant bed.

When inserting the final cup implant, the navigation system then displays the final inclination and anteversion values. The data generated during preparation of the implant bed and cup implantation are saved in a navigation system-dependent form. These data can be documented in surgery and treatment records. The procedure for implanting the prosthetic stem is not described here.

15.6 Conclusion and Future Perspectives

Ultrasound registration enables surgeons to achieve higher precision during the registration of bony landmarks in the anterior pelvic plane. As the bone surface is scanned directly, the surgeon can work independently of the overlying soft tissue layer. In heavily muscled obese men, this tissue layer is more likely to obstruct pointer palpation because it cannot be displaced or forced in as easily as in obese women, whose tissue is often softer. Similarly, the shape of the anterior superior iliac spine is not always sharply tapered and easily palpated with the pointer; to compensate for this, ultrasound registration can be used to search for identical topography of the iliac crest on both sides. This can be accomplished by always displaying the anterior inferior iliac spine on the same sectional plane.

In general, ultrasound is also very effective in visualizing the dorsal femoral condyles. An important element in shaft navigation, this plane is useful when defining shaft torsion. However, further developmental work is necessary in this regard to ensure secure horizontal alignment of the ultrasound transducer, since a slightly oblique plane would miss the dorsal culmination points of both femoral condyles.

Looking forward, developments such as automatic rapid landmark recognition (»intelligent ultrasound«) are envisaged for the future. Further conceivable applications would include registration in the lateral position and designs that connect commercial ultrasound devices to navigation systems, thereby saving costs. A long-term future goal could be to present image data on a tablet PC.

References

Hasart O, Perka C, Tohtz S (2008) Comparison Between Pointer-based and Ultrasound-based Navigation Technique in THA Using a Minimally Invasive Approach. Orthopedics 31 [10 Suppl 1]:31–34

Hasart O, Poepplau BM, Asbach P, Perka C, Wassilew GI (2009) Ultrasound-based navigation and 3D CT compared in acetabular cup position. Orthopedics 32 [10 Suppl]:6–10

Hirschmann MT, Affi FK, Helfrich C, Wirz D, Schwägli T, Overhoff HM, Moser W, Friederich NF (2011) Navigated total hip arthroplasty using a 3-D freehand ultrasound system: technical note and preliminary results. Orthopedics 34:816–820

Keppler P, Krysztoforski K, Swiatek E, Krowicki P, Kozak J, Gebhard F, Pinzuti JB (2007) A new experimental measurement and planning tool for sonographic-assisted navigation. Orthopedics 30 [10 Suppl]:S144–147

Kiefer H, Othman A (2007) Ultrasound vs pointer palpation based method in THA navigation: a comparative study. Orthopedics 30 [10 Suppl]:S153–156

Lee YS, Yoon TR (2008) Error in acetabular socket alignment due to the thick anterior pelvic soft tissues. J Arthroplasty 23:699–706

Parratte S, Kilian P, Pauly V, Champsaur P, Argenson JN (2008) The use of ultrasound in acquisition of the anterior pelvic plane in computer-assisted total hip replacement: a cadaver study. J Bone Joint Surg Br 90:258–263

Richolt JA, Rittmeister ME (2006) Misinterpretation of the anteversion in computer-assisted acetabular cup navigation as a result of a simplified palpation method of the frontal pelvic plane (in German). Z Orthop Ihre Grenzgeb 144:305–310

Spencer JM, Day RE, Sloan KE, Beaver RJ (2006) Computer navigation of the acetabular component: a cadaver reliability study.J Bone Joint Surg Br 88:972–975

Tretbar SH, Weiss EC, Hoss M, Schreiner S, Keppler P, Blömer W, Lemor RM (2002) Ultrasound hard tissue detection for registration in orthopedics and traumatology (in German). Biomed Tech (Berlin) 47 [Suppl 1 Pt 1]:434–437

Wassilew GI, Perka C, Janz V, König C, Asbach P, Hasart O (2012) Use of an ultrasound-based navigation system for an accurate acetabular positioning in total hip arthroplasty: a prospective, randomized, controlled study. Arthroplasty 27:687–69415

Process-Optimized Minimally Invasive Total Hip Replacement via a Direct Anterior Approach with Navigation Control of Leg Length and Offset[1]

Philipp Gebel, Markus Oszwald, Bernd Ishaque, Gaffar Ahmed, Recha Blessing, Fritz Thorey, Andreas Ottersbach

1 Competing interests: The development and production of the new leg positioner was realized by Condor Medicaltechnik, Salzkotten, Germany, while advice for the conception and for the clinical realization was mainly given by the orthopedic department in Brig. All patent and trademark rights lie entirely in the hands of Condor Medicaltechnik.

The purpose of this study was to analyze a new concept of using the minimally invasive direct anterior approach (DAA) in total hip replacement (THR) in combination with a leg positioner (Rotex-Table) and a modified retractor system (Condor). To control leg length and offset, the navigation system OrthoPilot® (B. Braun, Aesculap) or the Medacta system was used. We retrospectively evaluated the first 100 primary THRs performed with this new concept between 2009 and 2010, regarding the surgical data as well as the radiological and clinical outcome (Hip Disability and Osteoarthritis Outcome score, HOOS). All surgeries were perfomed following a standardized operation technique including navigation. The average age of the patients was 68 years (37–92 years), with a mean body mass index (BMI) of 26.5 (17–43).

The mean operating time was 80 min (55–130 min). There was an average blood loss of 511.5 ml (200–1,000 ml). No intraoperative complications occurred and the postoperative complication rate was 6%. The HOOS increased from 43 points preoperatively to 90 points (max. 100) 3 months after surgery. Radiological analysis showed an average cup inclination of 43° and a leg length discrepancy in the range of ±5 mm in 99% of cases.

This technique led to excellent clinic results, showed low complication rates, and in combination with navigation and an image intensifier allowed for correct implant positions while saving on manpower.

16.1 Materials and Methods

The initial results of the first 100 total hip replacements were analyzed. All patients were operated on using the DAA, in combination with the newly developed leg-positioning device and a modified retractor system (Condor Medicaltechnik, Salzkotten, Germany). All patients who underwent a total hip replacement between February 2009 and February 2010 with the process-optimized implantation method were included in the analysis. To objectify patient satisfaction and quality of surgery, the preoperative and the 3-month and 1-year postoperative outcomes were recorded using the Hip Disability and Osteoarthritis Outcome Score (HOOS). The postoperative conventional x-ray images were also evaluated in terms of cup inclination, lateralization, offset, and leg length. The inter-ischiacal line was used to measure cup inclination and leg length in comparison with the greater trochanter. Offset was defined as the distance center from the femoral head to the femoral stem axis. Lateralization was also measured from the caudal tip of the teardrop contour to the femoral stem axis (NIH 1994).

To estimate the outcome quality, the following factors were recorded: intraoperative blood loss, the type and frequency of complications, surgery time, time of hospitalization, and rehabilitation time.

16.1.1 Navigation Control

Two optoelectronic navigation systems were used to give the surgeon intraoperative control of leg length, lateralization of the femur, and measuring of offset. The open system of Medacta (Medacta, International SA, Strada Regina, Switzerland) was used to control offset and leg length when Medacta or Mathys products were implanted. All Aesculap prostheses were performed with the OrthoPilot® navigation system manufactured by B. Braun (B. Braun, Aesculap, Tuttlingen, Germany).

16.1.2 Ethics

The study presented was approved by the local ethics committee of Hannover Medical School, which follows the World Medical Association Declaration of Helsinki (nr. 917–2011).

16.1.3 Hip Osteoarthritis Outcome Score

The HOOS, first described in 2003 as an improvement to the widely used Western Ontario and MacMaster Universities Osteoarthritis Index (WOMAC), is a reliable and efficient tool for assessing total hip replacements (THRs) and has five relevant parameters: (a) *p*ain (P), (b) *s*ymptoms (S) – including impaired mobility and range of motion, (c) *a*ctivity limitation in daily living (A), (d) *sp*ort and recreation function (SP), and (d) hip-related *q*uality of life (Q) (min. 0 points, max. 100 points) (Nilsdotter et al. 2003; Ashby et al. 2008).

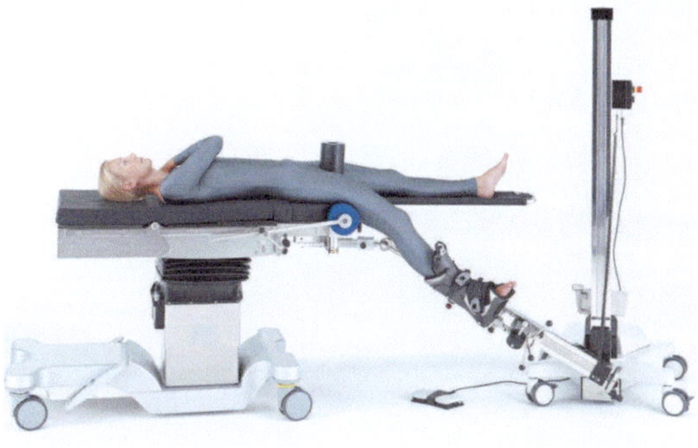

Fig. 16.1 Conventional fracture table (*left*) adapted with the Rotex-Table (*right*)

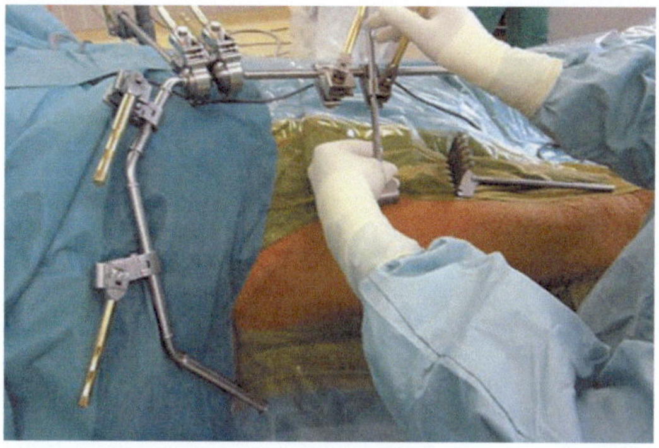

Fig. 16.2 Condor Gold Line-Retra

16.1.4 Patient Positioning with the Leg Positioner Rotex-Table

The newly developed Rotex-Table (Condor Medicaltechnik) is based on a vertical column, mounted on a mobile four-legged stand and connected to the extension table with an adapter mechanism (Fig. 16.1) The Rotex-Shoe is used to secure the extremity to be operated on with the system. This is the first positioner that has an anatomically beneficial design combining the use of quick-lock clips and carbon technology.

A motor drive, controlled by the surgeon with a foot pedal, is used to raise and lower the extremity. This function can also be applied using a switch mechanism manually on the column. For safety reasons, lowering and simultaneous extension of the extremity that can be set up via a thread pole is automatically blocked, so that extreme tissue stretching and the resulting nerve damage, for example, can be avoided. External rotation of the leg is manually set by the surgeon and automatically fixed in the desired position using a finely adjustable stop mechanism.

In practice, the patient's thigh is supported by an x-ray-permeable positioning roll positioned at the level of the picket between the patient's legs and about 3–5 cm above the table level. This positioning roll acts as a hypomochlion, to facilitate exposure of the proximal femur when the extremity is lowered. The healthy extremity is slightly abducted.

16.1.5 The Retractor System

The concept was adapted by adding a retractor system (Condor Medicaltechnik, Salzkotten, Germany) to further improve the intraoperative process. The system is secured to the extension bar of the operating table. A curved arm is applied in a cranial–lateral plane, and a straight bar is applied distally. The retractor system is aligned with the anterior superior iliac spine. Clamps are secured to both arms, to which the usual levers are later secured, ensuring an intraoperatively stable working position (Fig. 16.2).

16.1.6 Surgical Technique

An 8 cm skin incision is made 2–3 cm inferolateral to the anterior superior iliac spine following the course of the tensor fasciae latae muscle. The incision is made toward the fibula head. The subcutaneous tissue is then separated and the fascia of the tensor fasciae latae muscle opened and prepared between the tensor fasciae latae muscle and the rectus femoris muscle. Surrounding muscles and the cutaneus femoris lateralis nerve are preserved by a blunt preparation into the depth onto the capsule. The rectus femoris muscle is then pulled aside medially and the transverse branches of the femoral circumflex artery are clamped. After using the standard retractors that are connected to the condor system, the surgeon has a direct view of the ventral capsular structures of the hip joint. Three Hohmann

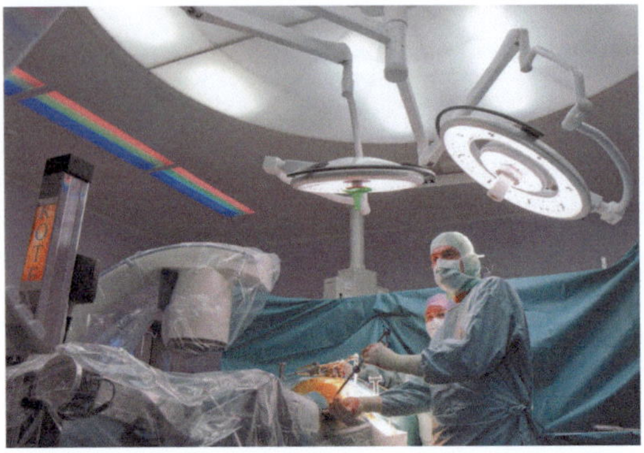

◘ **Fig. 16.3** Surgical set-up: combination of navigation and image intensifier

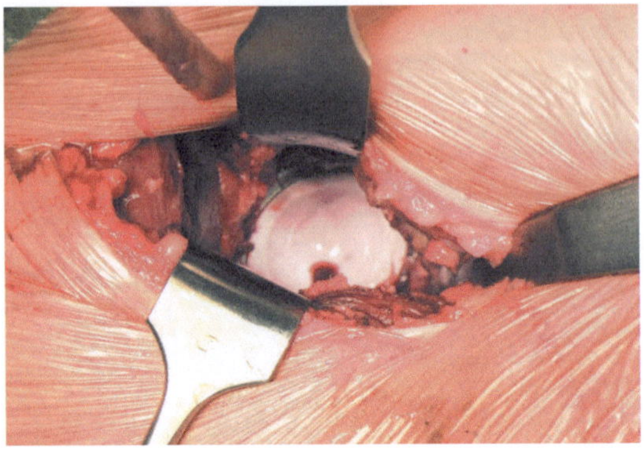

◘ **Fig. 16.4** Cup and inlay

retractors are used for good exposure of the anterior capsule. The ventral joint capsule is resected and the femoral neck is osteotomized at the planned level to remove the head. To expose the acetabulum, two retractors are applied to the medial and lateral acetabulum. After cup reaming to the planned size, the cup can be implanted using x-ray images and a navigation system (◘ Fig. 16.3 and ◘ Fig. 16.4)

To ensure adequate exposure of the femoral cavity, a step-by-step capsular release is performed. The surgeon initially sets the external rotation of the foot to about 90°, while receiving feedback on the tissue tension.

The capsular release is performed in three steps:

1. Electrical incision along the calcar to the lesser trochanter. The surgeon then carefully externally rotates the leg further.
2. Electrical incision in the extension of the osteotomized, dorsal femoral cortex to the medial boundary of the greater trochanter rotated medially in situ. The leg is then carefully further rotated externally by the surgeon and if necessary the release is extended. A bone hook is used to check if the proximal femur can be raised sufficiently. The greater trochanter must be able to slide at the acetabulum.
3. After slightly lowering the leg while pulling on the retractor on the femur and applying a retractor behind the greater trochanter, the third release in the region of the trochanteric fossa is performed vertical to the second release to free the dorsal capsule parts.

External rotation has to be extended from the final lowering of the leg to the preparation of the femur, until the tip of the osteotomized calcar corresponds at least to the sagittal axis of the patient and can even be positioned in slight external rotation.

The leg is now lowered with the motorized foot pedal control while pulling with the bone hook on the femur. The leg is lowered until internal rotation of the osteotomized level of the femur can be identified and the tip of the calcar is rotated medially over the patient's sagittal axis. The stem exposure can be supported by adducting the leg if necessary.

The femoral trial prosthesis can be easily repositioned following femoral preparation using the Rotex-table. The extended leg must not cause joint luxation at 90° external rotation.

The procedure described above for exposing the femoral cavity and subsequent reposition can be repeated swiftly using the Rotex-Table for implantation of the final prosthesis (◘ Fig. 16.5). These manipulations can be done by the surgeon without additional assistant staff.

After implantation the fascia and skin are closed. Patients are quickly mobilized with pain-adapted full weight bearing with underarm supports 1 day postoperatively.

16.1.7 Operating Staff

All THRs were carried out by a single surgeon with one medical assistant and one nurse.

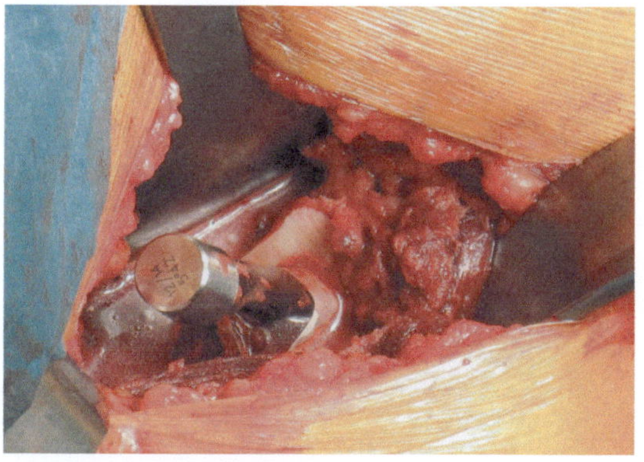

Fig. 16.5 Stem implantation

16.2 Results

The average age of the 50 women was 70.7 years (range, 51–92), and the average BMI was 26.4 (range, 17–43). The average age of the 50 men was 65.2 years (range, 37–84) and the BMI was 26.6 (range, 21–34). The surgical indication in 92 cases was primary osteoarthritis, there were four cases of femoral head necrosis, two cases of secondary osteoarthritis following proximal femur fracture, one case of femoral neck fracture, and one of dysplastic osteoarthritis (Tab. 16.1).

Different implants were used for THR (Tab. 16.2). The average operation time was 81 min (range, 55–130 min). Intraoperative blood loss was 511.5 ml on average (range, 200–1,000 ml). A cell saver was used in 80 cases. Eleven patients were given two erythrocyte concentrates each to treat postoperative anemia.

All patients were mobilized 1 day after surgery with underarm supports and full weight bearing permitted. After an average hospital stay of 8 days, all patients were independently mobile with walking sticks, and most were already able to walk a few steps without aids. Largely at the patient›s request, 31% of patients underwent follow-up treatment in a rehabilitation clinic following their hospital stay (Tab. 16.3).

The well-documented good clinical outcomes were also reflected in the high level of patient satisfaction. Evaluation of the HOOS at the 3-month follow-up averaged 90.96 points (value: S, P, A) and 89.59 (value: S, P, A, SP, Q). The values of category SP (sport and rehabilitation) reached 89.98 points and Q (quality of life) scored 85.02 points out of a total of 100. One year after surgery, the value slightly increased to 90.88 (value: S, P, A, SP, Q). Preoperatively, the average score was only 42.43 (value:

Tab. 16.1 Patient data

Hips (*n*)	100
Age (±SD, range)	68±11.8 years (37–92)
Gender (M/F; %m)	50
Side (right/left; % right)	56
Height (±SD, range)	169±8.7 cm (143–188)
Weight (±SD, range)	77±15.5 kg (45–115)
BMI (kg/m^2)	26.5±4.9 (17–43)
Navigated hips (%)	100
Preoperative diagnoses (5)	
Osteoarthritis	92
Dysplastic osteoarthritis	1
Avascular necrosis	4
Proximal femur fracture/ posttraumatic osteoarthritis	3

Tab. 16.2 Implants used

	Number of cases
Quadra-H, Versafit Cup, ceramic-on-ceramic, cementless (Medacta, Switzerland)	65
Metha short stem, PlasmaCup, ceramic-on-ceramic, cementless (B. Braun, Aesculap, Germany)	21
Excia stem, plasma cup, ceramic-on-ceramic, cementless (B. Braun, Aesculap, Germany)	4
Twinsys stem, Selexys Cup, ceramic-on-ceramic (Mathys, Germany)	8
Excia stem, PE cup, metal head (B. Braun, Aesculap, Germany)	2

Tab. 16.3 Operative data: clinical results

Operating time (±SD, range)	81±14.6 (55–130)
Navigated hips (%)	100
Cell saver (yes/no; % yes)	80
Estimated perioperative blood loss (±SD, range)	511.5±189 ml (200–1,000)
Postoperative transfusion of max. 2 erythrocyte concentrates (%)	11
Hospitalization time (±SD, range)	8.5±3.6 days (4–26)
Mobilization on crutches on 2nd postoperative day (%)	98
Mobilization on crutches during hospitalization time (%)	100
Rehabilitative follow-up treatment	31
HOOS preoperative (S, P, A)	42.43±14.6 (23.3–76)
HOOS 3 months postoperative (S, P, A, SP, Q) HOOS 1 year postoperative (S, P, A, SP, Q)	89.59±10.4 (49.4–100) 90.88±9.6 (52.8–100)

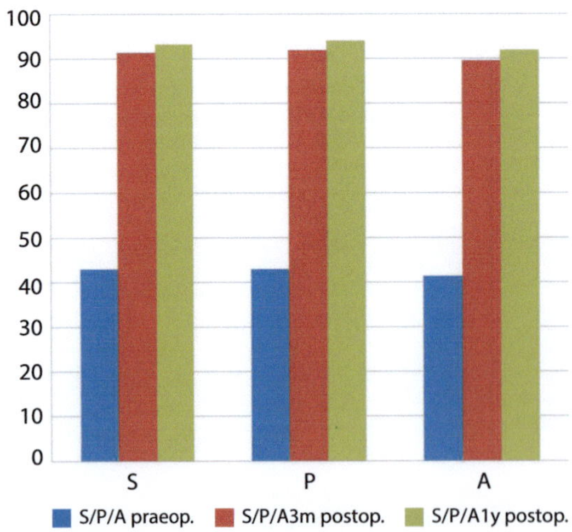

Fig. 16.6 Hip Osteoarthritis Outcome Score: preoperative (*blue column*), 3-month postoperative (*red column*), and 1-year (*green column*) postoperative points

Tab. 16.4 Complication rates

Intraoperative complications	0
Postoperative complications (%)	6
Reoperation rate (%)	2
Cup loosening	0
Stem loosening	0
Inlay fracture	1
Hip instability	1
Nerve irritations (Motor temporary/sensitivity persistent after 3 months)	2/1
Subsequent bleeding requiring revision surgery	0
Impaired wound healing	0
Venous thrombosis	1
Pulmonary embolism	0
Infection	0

S, P, A) out of a maximum score of 100; 85% of the postoperative questionnaires were available for evaluation (Fig. 16.6).

There were no intraoperative complications. Two patients had transient paresis of the femoral nerve. Another patient had an irritation of the lateral cutaneous femoral nerve. One case of recurrent dislocation was revised with an anterior approach, and successfully corrected by increasing the offset using the Merete system.

In one case, for an unexplained reason, the ceramic inlay fractured; this was successfully revised following the DAA. We observed one case of leg vein thrombosis despite prophylaxis with low-molecular-weight heparin. There were no further postoperative complications (Tab. 16.4)

All implantations were performed using navigation systems. Rigid body positioning, application of reference marks, and scanning of anatomical landmarks were successfully carried out via an anterior approach with the OrthoPilot® system from Aesculap and with the Medacta navigation system.

We also used an image converter to check the intraoperative positioning of the cup and stem. An

■ Tab. 16.5 Radiology results

Cup inclination (angle°)	43.2±4.36 (33–48)
Offset: preoperative/postoperative (mm) Difference in offset (postoperative–preoperative)	45.8/46.3 +1.26±4.97
Difference in lateralization Preoperative–postoperative (mm)	75/74 +0.04±5.90
Difference in leg length (%) [±5 mm (to −8 mm)]	99 (1)
Cup inclination (angle°)	43.2±4.36 (33–48)

ideal cup position was achieved in the majority of cases, as shown in the postoperative measurements on the conventional x-ray images. The cup inclination calculated from these results corresponded to the Lewinnek safe zone at an average of 43.2°, ±4.36 (33°–48°). There was no standardized measuring of the cup antetorsion. Leg length, lateralization, and offset were determined preoperatively and then postoperatively by measuring the x-ray images. The results were as follows: preoperative/postoperative offset, 45.8 mm/46.3 mm; preoperative/postoperative lateralization, 75 mm/74 mm.

Radiological measuring of leg length confirmed an almost equal length of both legs in 99 cases (difference of ±5 mm). There was only one case where a relevant difference of −8 mm to the other leg was found (■ Tab. 16.5).

16.3 Conclusion

The aim of our study was to analyze the new concept of using a minimally invasive direct anterior approach (DAA) in THR in combination with a leg positioner (Rotex-Table), a modified retractor system (Condor), and navigation systems to control leg length and offset. Furthermore, we wanted to evaluate the efficiency and the ergonomic and financial effectiveness of our procedure.

For a good surgical outcome, it is important to standardize the working processes and to facilitate the much-criticized difficult exposure of the proximal femur in the DAA. This was achieved by developing and using the Rotex-Table and systematic release techniques as well as by using an adapted retractor system. Apart from significantly simplifying the process, we have also succeeded in developing a standardized operation sequence, where it has been possible to reduce costs by eliminating the need for the assistant and positioning staff without having a negative impact on the quality of treatment.

As our clinical observations on the first 100 patients illustrate, process-optimized hip replacement via DAA and with control of leg length and offset by navigation results in great patient satisfaction and low complication rates as well as in excellent implant positioning.

References

Ashby E, Grocott MPW, Haddad FS (2008) Outcome measures for orthopaedic interventions on the hip. J Bone Joint Surg Br 90:545–549

Nilsdotter AK, Lohmander LS, Klässbo M, Roos EM (2003) Hip disability and osteoarthritis outcome score (HOOS)-validity and responsiveness in total hip replacement. BMC Musculoskeletal Disorders 4:10

NIH (1994) Consensus Statement, Total Hip Replacement. Sept. 12-14; Vol.12, no. 5

Navigation in Trauma Surgery

Multidepartmental Use of a Fixed 3D Navigation System

Florian Gebhard, Bastian Scheiderer, Peter Richter, Christoph Riepl

In principle, navigation in trauma surgery involves two procedures.

Two-dimensional (2D) navigation is based on two regular fluoroscopic images and copies that are transferred to the navigation system. Instruments can be visualized in a maximum of three different projections at a time.

Three-dimensional (3D) navigation is an enhancement of 2D navigation and requires computed tomography (CT)-like data. Two alternative pathways can be used: first, intraoperative matching of a preoperative CT scan; second, performing an intraoperative 3D scan. The latter is usually registered automatically.

3D navigation has emerged as the best choice in pelvic and spinal surgery (Raftopoulos et al. 2012) as well as in surgery of the large joints. A limitation so far is the displayed field of view. A conventional C-arm system creates a cubic data set with an edge length of 13.5 cm (Arcadis© Orbic 3D, Siemens, Germany). Flat-panel detectors enable a larger display window and are currently used in new angiographic systems.

One such system is the Artis zeego system (Siemens). In comparison to other angiography systems, the Artis zeego C-arm is held by a robotic guidance system. The fluoroscopy unit, which rotates around the patient, is fixed to the robotic arm. It is equipped with a flat-panel detector. Therefore, the Artis zeego system can generate a significantly larger display window in a single scan.

In this system the fluoroscope is connected to the operating table, which allows for simultaneous movement of the table and the C-arm. The latter is important for storage of image position and to prevent collision. The DynaCT function provides a CT-like image that has good soft tissue and bone contrast. In addition, the Artis zeego system has the classic characteristics of an angiography device. Recently, the authors introduced a link to a navigation unit (Brainlab Curve™ system).

17

It was a substantial challenge to integrate a navigation system into this predefined setting. Over a process of several years, the authors and the participating companies Siemens and Brainlab developed a setting that made navigation in a robotic C-arm system possible.

The latest 3D navigation software is used (Spine 3.0®, Brainlab, Germany) in the new Curve™ system (Brainlab). This system enables optimal data acquisition owing to the larger camera range and angle of view. This setting could be realized with the construction of the new center of surgery at Ulm University (Fig. 17.1).

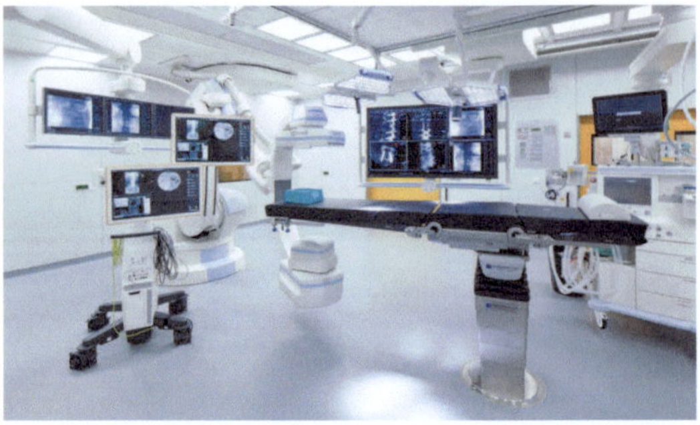

Fig. 17.1 Operating room set-up for computer-assisted 3D image-guided surgery

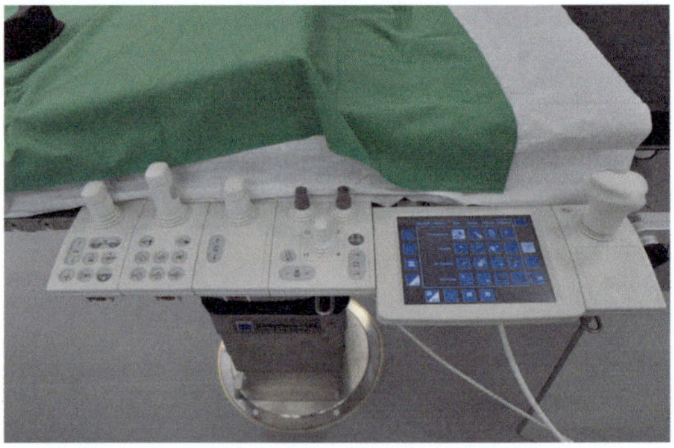

Fig. 17.2 Control panel at the OR table

17.1 Materials and Methods

A control unit is used to steer the system comprising the robotic fluoroscopy unit and the operating room (OR) table (Fig. 17.2)

In the intraoperative setting the patient lies on a carbon fiber table, which is physically connected to the C-arm according to the room position.

The imaging system has a memory function that permits important projections that are used during the operation procedure to be saved. These images are taken in a nonsterile setting, where the patient is already placed on the table (Fig. 17.3a–c).

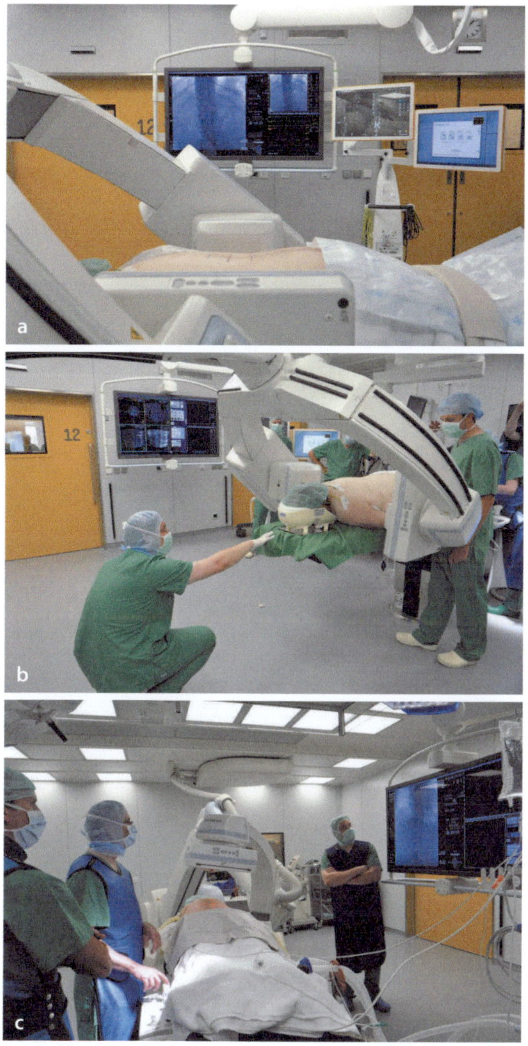

Fig. 17.3 Determination and storage of the lateral position (**a**); collision check (**b**); determination and storage of the oblique position (**c**)

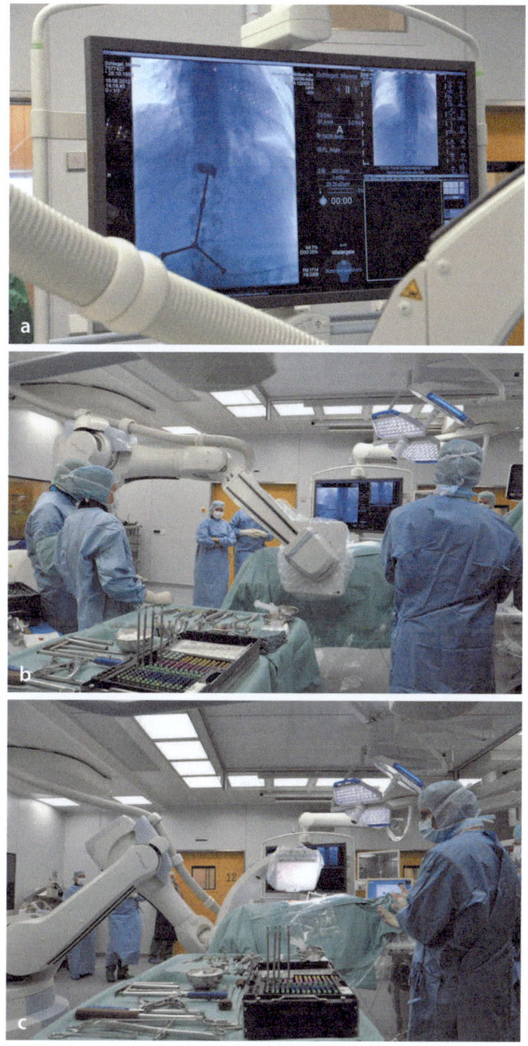

Fig. 17.5 Data referencing base check (**a**), preparation for the 3D scan (**b**), performing the 3D scan. It is important to clear the distance to the C-arm (**c**)

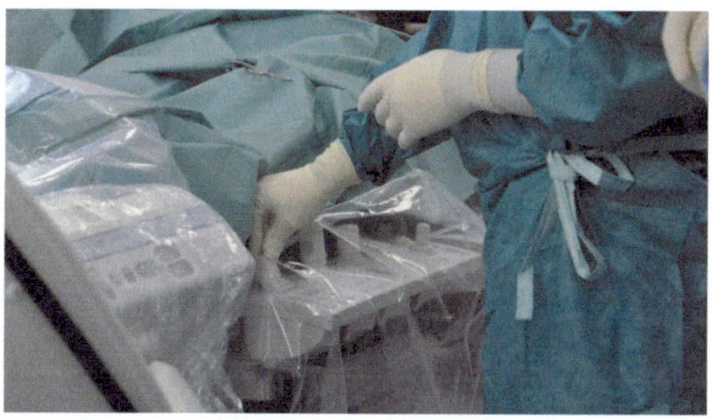

Fig. 17.4 Sterile cover of the control unit

Subsequently, the operation starts by placing the sterile covering. Angiographic covers with a transparent sheet are used, allowing free access to the control panel (Fig. 17.4)

The control panel allows the surgeon to control the imaging for the entire duration of the operation.

After checking the initially adjusted fluoroscopy positions, standard surgical procedures begin with the fixation of the data referencing base (DRB) and a check of the position with respect to interference with the subsequent scan (Fig. 17.5a). The differ-

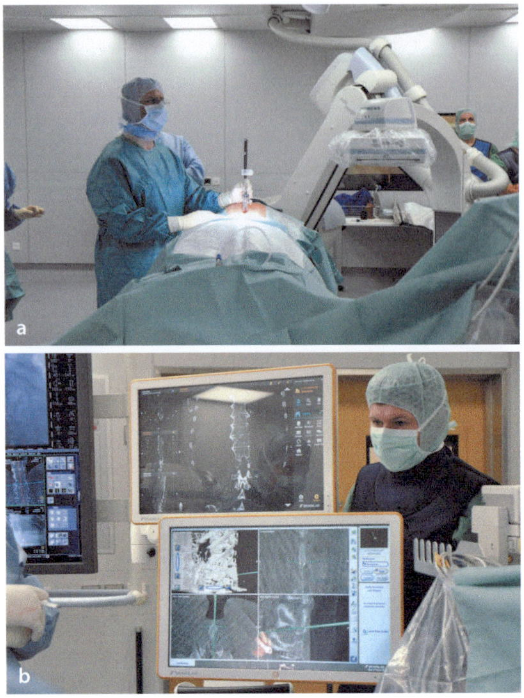

Fig. 17.6 Accuracy check (**a**) and displayed accuracy check (**b**)

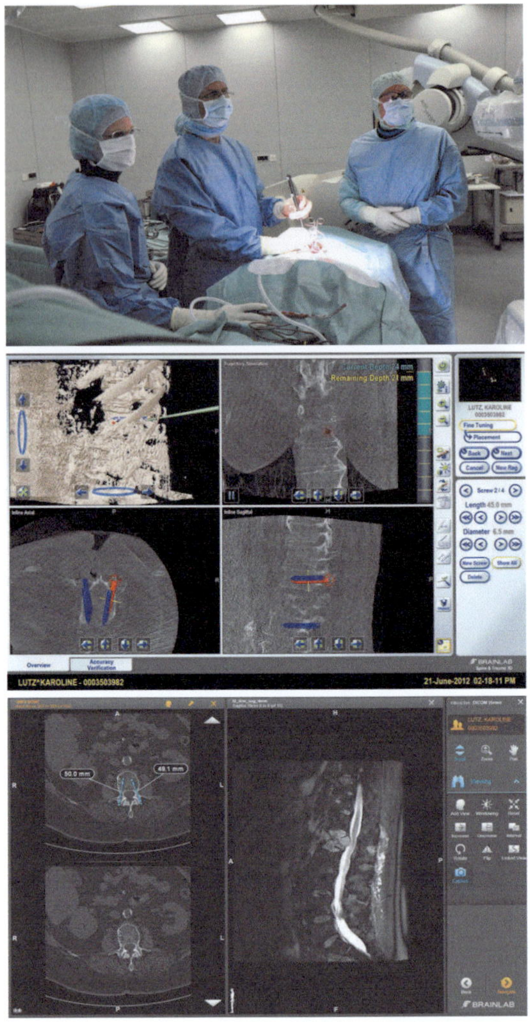

a

b

c

Fig. 17.7 Screw planning (**a**), automatic screw check (**b**), and comparison with the preoperative planning (**c**)

ent end positions of the system are then automatically started and the image acquisition is tested (Fig. 17.5b).

At this point, corrections to the height and position of the table in relation to the C-arm may be necessary.

By using a pointer-based remote control for CAS and joysticks for the fluoroscopy unit, the C-arm and the navigation system can be handled from the sterile operating table without the need for sterile covering of monitors and similar equipment.

After a successful test run, a 190° scan is performed within seconds providing a 3D data set of 270 images (Fig. 17.5c). The data set is automatically registered and transferred to the navigation system. After the gray-scale setting has been adapted, the data set can be used for navigation immediately.

The imaging is followed by a standard navigation work-flow starting with an accuracy check (Fig. 17.6a,b), which, however, differs from the conventional procedure as there is a larger field of view available (Fig. 17.7b).

With respect to the spine, this means that at least eight to ten vertebral bodies can be displayed on one image section and that a simultaneous pedicle screw planning (Fig. 17.7a,b) can be performed for all affected vertebral bodies simultaneously. The planned screws can be compared with the preoperatively planned ones that are simultaneously displayed by one of the two monitors of the CAS systems (Fig. 17.7c).

However, the standard preventative safety measures are to be maintained, for example, the distance to the DRB and the motion of the DRB or the patient.

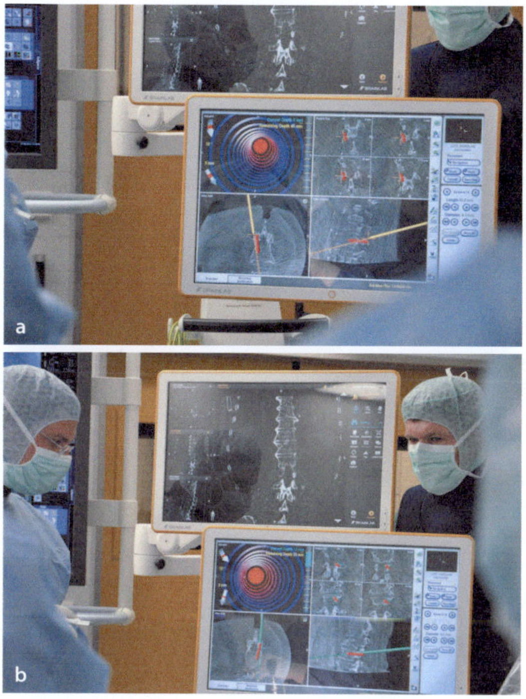

■ **Fig. 17.8a,b** Screw placement I (**a**); screw placement II (b)

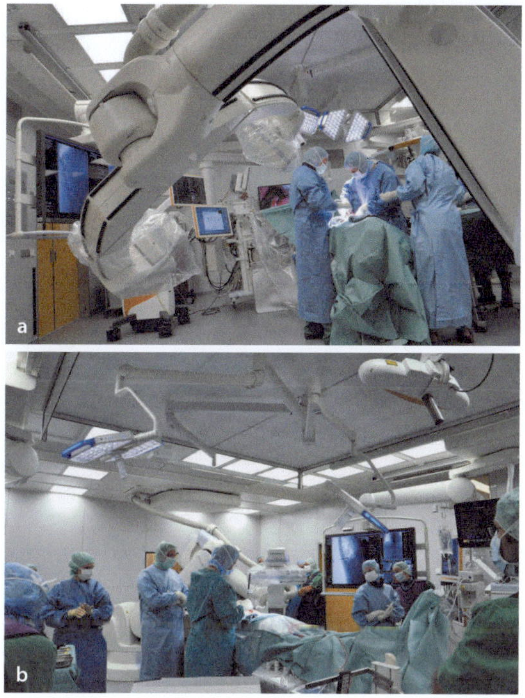

■ **Fig. 17.9a,b** Performing surgery with the C-arm in a parking position

17.2 Results

Since implementing the system, 14 spinal procedures were performed within the first 4 weeks. These ranged from cases of bisegmental to multisegmental stabilizations. All navigation steps carried out with this system were failure-free and all pedicle screws were placed correctly (■ Fig. 17.8a,b).

At any time point during the surgery, the fluoroscopy unit can be put in a parking position and recalled quickly and precisely (■ Fig. 17.9a,b).

Owing to the high image quality, a second round of CT scanning is performed after pedicle screw insertion intraoperatively; in the case of minimally invasive surgery, it is performed after the insertion of guide pins to ensure correct placement.

Since the image quality of the fluoroscopy scan is comparable to that of the standard postoperative CT scan, it can serve as a postoperative examination of the final screw positioning. A transfer to the PACS system is possible.

In general, the system distinguishes itself in that it can be handled intuitively by the surgeon. However, appropriate training and instruction, especially for the robotic C-arm system and the operating table, are essential.

17.3 Conclusion

The system discussed in this chapter offers the highest resolution and accuracy for 3D navigation currently available, with the advantage of allowing intraoperative registered datasets to be generated and thereby eliminating the challenges posed by matching.

Both systems, the fluoroscopy unit as well as the CAS system, are high-end solutions in their field and require the corresponding training.

After careful preparation and thorough training in patient positioning, C-arm control, and navigation, experienced surgeons can implement this system. The image quality is outstanding. Even for obese patients (>120 kg) with corresponding soft tissue interference, high-quality images that are free of artifacts can be generated.

Justification for the acquisition of such a high-cost operating room is that it can also serve other surgical specialties such as cardiac surgery or neurosurgery. In cardiac surgery, the system is used for minimally invasive valve replacement since it offers 3D vessel reconstructions as well as planning and targeting of the correct stent position. For neurosurgery, the system has the advantage of allowing angiography of cranial aneurysms to be performed in combination with CAS including an integrated high-end microscope (Pentero©, Zeiss, Germany).

Reference

Raftopoulos C, Waterkeyn F, Fomekong E, Duprez T (2012) Percutaneous pedicle screw implantation for refractory low back pain: from manual 2D to fully robotic intraoperative 2D/3D fluoroscopy. Tech Stand Neurosurg 38:75–93

3D Navigation with a Mobile C-arm

Jochen Franke, Paul Alfred Grützner

In the field of imaging-assisted navigation, three-dimensional (3D) navigation with a mobile C-arm currently represents the gold standard in trauma surgery in terms of flexibility and mobility, and can now also be deployed rapidly and in a more user-friendly manner in changing anatomical situations. It has been in routine use for 10 years at several centers in the treatment of spinal and pelvic injuries, as well as in the foot and ankle joint region.

The technique of image data acquisition and 3D navigation with the Arcadis Orbic 3D (Siemens AG, Erlangen, Germany) and the navigation system Navivision (Brainlab AG, Feldkirchen, Germany) will be briefly described as an example. In addition to the C-arm and the navigation system integrated in the trolley of the C-arm, the system requires an optoelectronic camera on a mobile, lightweight support. The additional monitor of the navigation system is mounted on the trolley. The patient has to be positioned on a radiolucent carbon fiber table. With the mobile 3D C-arm, a 3D-volume image dataset with an edge length of approximately 12 cm is produced from 100 individual projections during a scan through a 190° orbital rotation around the object (patient). A reference base has to be fixed on the object (attached at the bone) beforehand. Registration is done automatically at the beginning of the scan. The 3D dataset is then also transmitted automatically through an interface to the navigation unit. The computer-assisted surgery can now be performed with (pre-)calibrated instruments in the corresponding segment of the volume image dataset. The practicability and results of 3D navigation with a mobile C-arm will be demonstrated with reference to the literature. The presentation is organized according to anatomical regions and the main indications are described for these regions.

18.1 Spine

18.1.1 Pedicle Screw Placement in the Thoracic and Lumbar Spine

18

The main goal of navigation on the thoracic and lumbar spine (◘ Fig. 18.1, Fig. 18.2, Fig. 18.3, Fig. 18.4) is to improve the accuracy of pedicle screw placement. These endeavors were motivated not least by reports in the literature of malpositioning of pedicle screws in a high percentage of cases: in up to 30% of cases for the lumbar spine and in up to 55% for the thoracic spine (Gertzbein and Robbins 1990; Tjardes et al. 2010). The precision of computer navigation-assisted pedicle instrumentation has been investigated in numerous experimental and clinical studies. The misplacement rates were in some cases reported to be in the very low range of between 0% and 8% (Grützner et al. 2004; Wendl et al. 2003). Generally, however, an inconsistent picture emerges not only for computed tomography (CT)- or fluoroscopy-based navigation, but also for mobile 3D C-arm-assisted navigation. A comparative study of screws introduced using a navigated versus a non-navigated technique showed a considerable improvement in accuracy accompanied by a markedly shorter fluoroscopy time in favor of navigation (Wendl et al. 2003). Another study that compared 3D with 2D navigation, however, found no significant differences (Lekovic et al. 2007). Meta-analyses show that with navigation, better results tend to be obtained for the lumbar spine and the thoracolumbar transition, but not for the thoracic spine (Tjardes et al. 2010). This is surprising, especially considering that navigation should be particularly advantageous in the thoracic spine because of the smaller pedicle diameter and the worse image quality in this region.

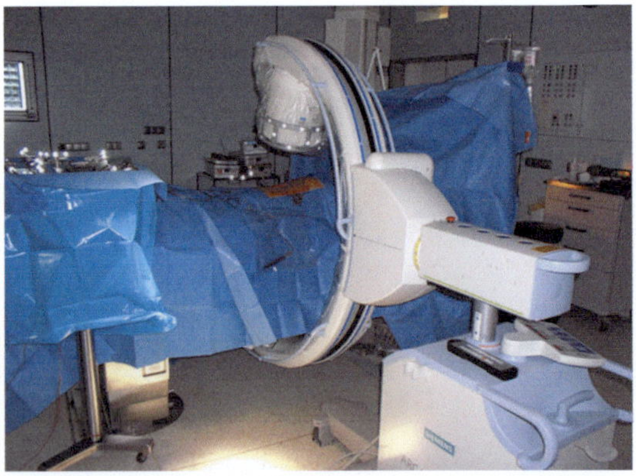

◘ **Fig. 18.1** Set-up for computer-assisted pedicle instrumentation. The camera is at the end of the foot. The operating area can be covered with sterile drapes for the scan. The reference base protrudes through a hole cut into a drape. After the scan, the drape is cut in the middle and drops down on both sides (not shown)

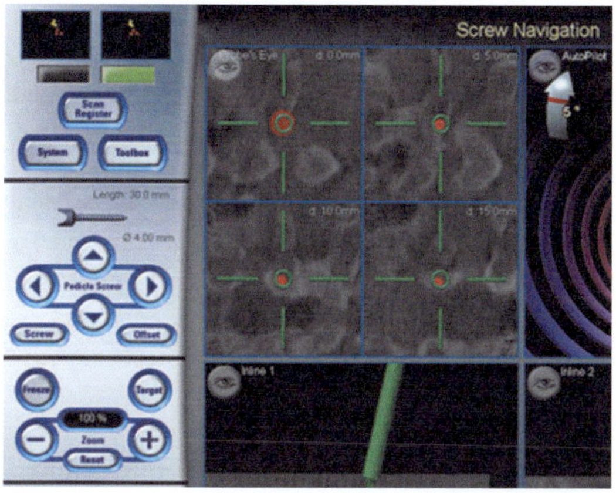

Fig. 18.2 Computer-assisted opening of the pedicle with the pedicle probe after preoperative screw planning

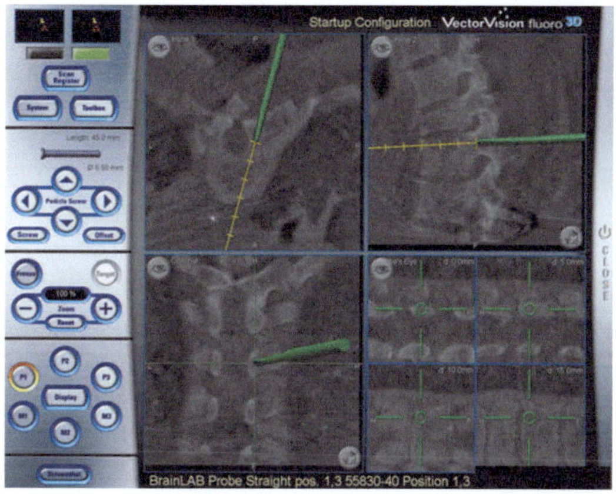

Fig. 18.3 Computer-assisted preparation of the screw channel with the pedicle awl

An analysis of the problems associated with misplaced pedicle screws following the introduction of navigation has shown not only that study designs frequently differ, but also that there is no uniform definition of the term »misplaced« (Kosmopoulos and Schizas 2007). This is naturally a major obstacle to interpreting and comparing different studies. It is equally difficult to define the importance of misplacement at all, and from what degree onward misplacement has clinical consequences. Experience has shown that most medial or lateral perforations of a pedicle are without clinical consequences and are only noticed on postoperative CT scans (Wendl et al. 2011).

Another aspect concerns the heterogeneous patient samples. Many studies derive their data from patient populations including subjects with degenerative diseases (Schleicher et al. 2009), and for the reasons outlined above the data concerned cannot invariably be extrapolated to the situation existing in trauma care.

Almost all investigations have shown, however, that even computer navigation offers no guarantee that misplacements will be avoided.

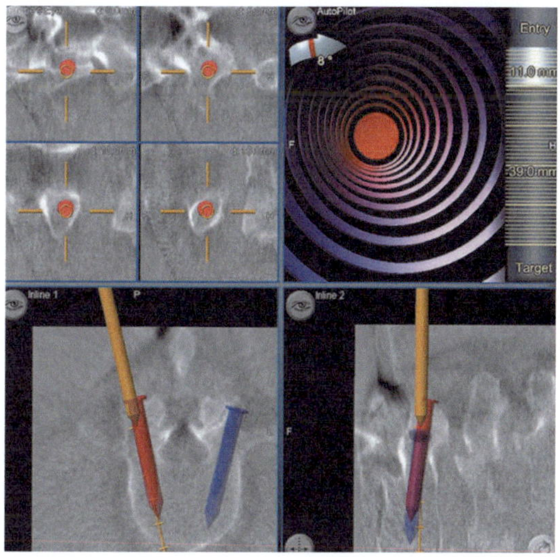

Fig. 18.4 Computer-assisted pedicle screw placement after bilateral planning

18.1.2 Radiation Exposure

One undisputed advantage of navigation is that it reduces exposure to radiation. The dorsal instrumentation of pedicles is associated with a relatively high exposure to x-rays. This applies both for the patients and the operating theater personnel. Several studies on this topic have shown that navigation leads to a marked reduction in radiation exposure. The particular advantage of intraoperative 3D fluoroscopy for the surgical team lies in the fact that the team can leave the control area during the scan and is therefore not subject to any additional radiation exposure (Grützner et al. 2004; Wendl et al. 2003).

18.1.3 Time Requirement

Navigation takes time, both pre- and intraoperatively. An increase in the operating time is to be expected especially during the initial learning curve (Schleicher et al. 2009). A special challenge is presented by emergency situations, in which a team experienced in navigation is not available. The sometimes considerable time required for preoperative planning and intraoperative matching when using CT datasets, however, is drastically reduced when using mobile 3D C-arm navigation.

18.1.4 Financial Aspects

Watkins et al. have addressed the question as to how 3D C-arm-assisted navigation in the thoracic and lumbar spinal region rates with regard to financial aspects (Watkins et al 2010). In their study they compared 100 consecutive patients with computer-assisted pedicle screw placement with a historical, conventionally treated control group. They based their calculation on the costs of the revision surgeries performed to correct screw misplacements (3% conventional, 0% navigated). They concluded that a reduction in the total costs can result when a large number of surgeries are performed. Projecting their calculation against their reported costs of the navigation equipment, amortization would already be achieved with 20 revision operations rendered unnecessary. The implementation of a navigation system with a 3D C-arm generates costs of around € 400,000. Depending on the reimbursement system, it is at best doubtful whether this would be the case in most countries, including Germany.

18.1.5 Screw Placement in the Cervical Spine

The cervical spine is to be regarded as a high-risk area in terms of pedicle instrumentation. The anatomical structures are small, and the vertebral artery running close to the vertebral body is an additional risk factor. The corridor for the safe placement of screws is therefore very narrow on the cervical spine. In addition to pedicle instrumentations, navigated transarticular C1/C2 screw placements via the Magerl technique and transpedicular C2 screw osteosyntheses have been described (Hott et al. 2004; Rajasekaran et al. 2007). Although the technical practicability has been demonstrated in studies, no conclusive evidence of an advantage of navigation has yet been presented (Tjardes et al. 2010)]. Elsewhere, however, a trend toward a reduced rate of screw misplacements has been demonstrated, especially under confined anatomical conditions (Hott et al. 2004; Ito et al. 2007).

The secure fixation of the dynamic reference base (DRB) on the spine is technically demanding. Moreover, the mobility of the cervical spine is much greater than that of the thoracolumbar spine, and a DRB on the adjacent vertebra can more rapidly result in inaccuracies. In summary, navigation on the cervical spine has been introduced at only a few specialized centers where it has been used in studies or experimentally. Despite the potential advantages described, it is still a long way from being introduced into clinical routine.

18.2 Pelvis

18.2.1 Sacroiliac Screw Placement

Screw placement in the posterior pelvic ring for injuries of the sacroiliac joint is technically demanding because of the complex anatomy, the narrow corridor for the screws, and the vulnerable soft tissues surrounding them (nerves, vessels). In the conventional procedure, fluoroscopy times of up to 10 min per screw have been reported (Stöckle et al. 2007). With the navigated technique, first the correct site of entry is marked on the skin with the pointer. Following blunt dissection and identification of the point of entry on the bone, a Kirschner wire is introduced transversely into the sacroiliac joint using a navigated drill guide (■ Fig. 18.5). It should be noted here that the Kirschner wire has a certain flexibility and may possibly take a different direction than intended. In cases of doubt, the result can be checked with a repeat 3D scan. After correct placement, the wire is overdrilled and the cannulated screw is introduced. With soft bone, the drilling operation can be left out. If the risk of wire mis-

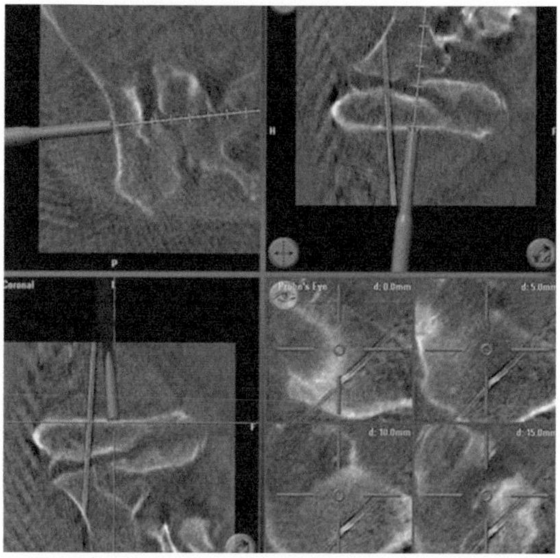

Fig. 18.5 Placement of the Kirschner wire with the navigated drill guide

placement because of its flexibility is to be avoided, drilling can also be carried out directly.

The advantage of 3D navigation is not only the better orientation it provides, but also the superior visualization of the region. This is less helpful in fluoroscopy, which is necessary for both the conventional procedure and for 2D navigation. Although 3D-CT-based navigation offers the best image quality, it involves the demanding and error-prone process of matching. In addition, nothing must have changed in the meantime in the anatomical conditions, otherwise considerable inaccuracies are to be expected. For these reasons, 3D navigation with the C-arm has become the favored navigation technique at most centers. Nevertheless, publications in the literature confine themselves to small case numbers. A trend toward a lower misplacement rate compared to all other techniques is discernible (Stöckle et al. 2007; Grützner et al. 2002; König et al. 2011).

18.2.2 Minimally Invasive Screw Placement at the Acetabulum

In surgical management, acetabular fractures are usually treated by open reduction and internal fixation. In some patients, however, the fracture morphology allows for percutaneous minimally invasive screw osteosynthesis. This is only possible with nondislocated, simple fractures that do not require reduction. Even slightly dislocated fractures that can be reduced by percutaneous manipulation with, for example, a Schanz screw are accessible to minimally invasive osteosynthesis. The anatomy of the acetabulum is complex, the corridor for screw placement often narrow. Therefore it is a challenge for surgeons and especially for their 3D spatial sense. Navigation is thus the ideal solution under these conditions. In various laboratory trials, 3D fluoroscopy navigation was shown to provide greater accuracy compared to 2D fluoroscopy navigation and to the conventional non-navigated technique (Gras et al. 2012; Ochs et al. 2010). The practicability and accuracy of the method have already been confirmed not only in laboratory trials, but also in clinical use (Hong et al. 2010; Lin et al. 2008). 3D navigation can also be used in the open surgical procedure. Following reduction and temporary Kirschner wire osteosynthesis of the fragments, a 3D scan can be helpful in checking the reduction quality. If a reference base is attached to the bone beforehand, the image data can additionally be used for navigated screw placement (König et al. 2011). The risk of intra-articular screw placement is thereby reduced.

18.3 Foot and Ankle

18.3.1 Retrograde Drilling of Talar Osteochondral Lesions

Retrograde navigated drilling of osteochondritis dissecans tali, like minimally invasive screw placement in the pelvis, is an outstanding example of how the surgeon is shown the way via the 3D visualization supported by the navigation system. Orientation presents a challenge particularly because the direction of drilling in the talus in all planes does not follow any anatomical reference. This situation is made even more difficult by the fact that the lesions sometimes have a diameter of hardly more than 5–6 mm. This is illustrated by individual reports of lesions that have not been reached or have been missed (Richter and Zech 2011); the unreported figure could be high. The decisive advantage of mobile 3D navigation is the immediate possibility of verifying the result. In our own procedure, first the diagnosis and the intact state of the overlying cartilage are confirmed arthroscopically. The dynamic reference base must be fixed in the neck of the talus and thus in the scanning field in such a way that it neither impedes navigation with artifacts nor leads to collisions with the consecutively used instruments. After the 3D scan, a drilling wire can be placed using navigated drill guides. A repeat 3D scan is performed to check that the tip of the wire is also definitely touching the lesion as centrally as possible. The site is then drilled open stepwise from 4.5 mm to 6 mm and to a maximum of 8 mm under fluoroscopic control and the canal is filled with an autologous bone grafting from the iliac crest. If necessary, the final result can now be checked again by 3D scanning and can be documented. The technical effort involved is high, but so is the safety for the patient and surgeon. The procedure is minimally invasive and very soft-tissue sparing. Other working groups have described a similar surgical procedure (Richter and Zech 2010; Geerling et al. 2009b; Kendoff et al. 2003). Comparisons based on, for example, operating and fluoroscopy time, precision, and definitively successful drilling in relation to the selected workflow do not exist in the literature. Compared with direct drilling, initial wire placement has the advantage that if the lesion is not contacted centrally, the wire can be angulated toward the center of the lesion after the first and possibly also after the second drilling. In this way, slight deviations in the initial wire placement can be compensated. Initial short-term results suggest that, overall, the demanding procedure could be justified. After a mean follow-up of 25 months, significant improvements in clinical scores and a high rate of revascularizations visible on magnetic resonance images of areas of previously impaired blood flow were reported (Geerling et al. 2009b).

18.3.2 Screw Placement at the Calcaneus

The use of intraoperative 3D imaging in the surgical management of calcaneus fractures has now become a routine procedure at many centers. This is because of the high intraoperative revision rates after 3D imaging, which have already been reported in several publications (Geerling et al. 2009a; Rübberdt et al. 2006; Rammelt et al. 2002). Geerling and colleagues reported a revision rate of 41% in 2009. The study, however, included only 32 patients (Geerling et al. 2009a). The largest patient sample published to date comprised 82 subjects. In 14.6% of cases, a screw correction and in 7.3% correction of the reduction of the posterior joint facet were performed (Rübberdt et al. 2006). Various authors have shown that up to two-thirds of posterior joint facets cannot be reliably assessed by conventional fluoroscopy in the standard projections (Rübberdt et al. 2006; Rammelt et al. 2002). This is the main reason why implant malpositions and residual steps and gaps of the articular surfaces are regularly overlooked.

Other research groups have also determined rates of between 6% and 25% for misplaced screws in calcaneal osteosynthesis (Rübberdt et al. 2006; Richter et al. 2005). Up to 20% of these affected the sustentacular screws, which were either positioned intra-articularly in the lower ankle joint or did not secure the sustentacular fragment. Causally responsible for this high misplacement rate is the lack of prominent anatomical starting points and the oblique course of the sustentacular screws directly below the convexly shaped posterior joint surface (Rübberdt et al. 2006; Richter et al. 2005; Kienast et al. 2006). Several groups have used 3D navigation to improve the precision of sustentacular screw placement (Rübberdt et al. 2009; Gras et al. 2010). One group placed 20 screws in 15 calcanei with the navigated technique and checked the result by 3D scan. All the screws were found to be in the intended position. As a result, the operating time increased by a mean 11.9 min (±2.2 min) (Rübberdt et al. 2009). In another trial, eight sustentacular screws per group were introduced into artificial bone (synbone). Three different navigation techniques were compared with conventional, non-navigated screw placement. CT was used to assess the actual screw position. No significant differences in the accuracy of screw placement were detected. However, an additional fluoroscopy time of 17 s (±1.03 s) was noted in the 2D fluoroscopy navigation group and of 66.8 s (±0.9 s) in the 3D fluoroscopy navigation group.

The mean time to screw placement was reported as 13.32 min (±0.49 min) in the 2D navigation group, as 19.04 min (±1.41 min) in the 3D navigation group, as 3.49 min (±0.26 min) in the fluoroscopy-free navigation group, and as a mere 1.26 min (±0.05 min) in the conventional group (Gras et al. 2010). Although it was concluded that navigation appears to be helpful and that 3D navigation provides the best orientation, the question must nevertheless be asked whether the high investment of time, material, and radiation exposure is justified by the benefits. Certainly, this will most likely be the case in minimally invasive percutaneous screw osteosynthesis of the calcaneus.

18.4 Summary and Outlook

The indications presented here are those for which 3D navigation with a mobile C-arm is regularly used at the centers concerned. Its use in other anatomical regions is rare and is more experimental. Based on our own experience, however, this type of navigation is helpful in many regions, from navigated Magerl screw placement in the cervical spine, to navigated kypho- or vertebroplasty, to navigated drilling of an osteoid osteoma of the calcaneus. The first step has been taken with the integration of the navigation system into the trolley of the C-arm. In the interest of more widespread use, however, greater user-friendliness is called for. The systems must be intuitive and easy to use, offer great accuracy and thus patient safety, and must become easy in hardware handling. Moreover, integrating the system into the operating room would offer great advantages for surgery preparation and space management. Recent developments and the installation of the first hybrid operating rooms are moving precisely in this direction. Some time is likely to pass, however, before a noteworthy number is available for use in traumatology.

References

Geerling J, Kendoff D, Citak M, Zech S, Gardner MJ, Hüfner T, Krettek C, Richter M (2009a) Intraoperative 3D imaging in calcaneal fracture care-clinical implications and decision making. J Trauma 66:768–773

Geerling J, Zech S, Kendoff D, Citak M, O'Loughlin PF, Hüfner T, Krettek C, Richter M (2009b) Initial outcomes of 3-dimensional imaging-based computer-assisted retrograde drilling of talar osteochondral lesions. Am J Sports Med 37:1351–1357

Gertzbein SD, Robbins SE (1990) Accuracy of pedicular screw placement in vivo. Spine 15:11–14

Gras F, Marintschev I, Wilharm A, Lindner R, Klos K, Mückley T, Hofmann GO (2010) Sustentaculum tali screw placement for calcaneus fractures – different navigation procedures compared to the conventional technique (in German). Z Orthop Unfall 148:309–318

Gras F, Marintschev I, Klos K, Mückley T, Hofmann GO, Kahler DM (2012) screw placement for acetabular fractures; which navigation modality (2-dimensional vs. 3-dimensional) should be used? An experimental study. J Orthop Trauma [Epub ahead of print]

Grützner PA, Rose E, Vock B, Holz F, Nolte LP, Wentzensen A (2002) Computer assisted percutaneous transileosacral screw osteosynthesis. Experiences with a passive optoelectronic navigation system based on precalibrated fluoroscopic images. Unfallchirurg 105:254–260

Grützner PA, Beutler T, Wendl K et al (2004) Intraoperative three-dimensional navigation for pedicle screw placement (in German). Chirurg 75:967–975

Hong G, Cong-Feng L, Cheng-Fang H, Chang-Qing Z, Bing-Fang Z (2010) Percutaneous screw fixation of acetabular fractures with 2D fluoroscopy-based computerized navigation. Arch Orthop Trauma Surg 130:1177–1783

Hott JS, Papadopoulos SM, Theodore N, Dickman CA, Sonntag VK (2004) Intraoperative Iso-C C-arm navigation in cervical spinal surgery: review of the first 52 cases. Spine 29:2856–2860

Ito H, Neo M, Yoshida M et al (2007) Efficacy of computer-assisted pedicle screw insertion for cervical instability in RA patients. Rheumatol Int 27:567–574

Kendoff D, Geerling J, Mahlke L, Citak M, Kfuri M Jr, Hüfner T, Krettek C (2003) Navigated Iso-C(3D)-based drilling of a osteochondral lesion of the talus (in German). Unfallchirurg 106:963–967

Kienast B, Gille J, Queitsch C, Kaiser MM, Thietje R, Juergens C, Schulz AP (2006) Improved therapy of calcaneal fractures by intraoperative 3d-fluoroscopy and locked-screw plate fixation. Eur J Trauma 32:471–476

König B, Freude T, Schäffler A, Ochs BG, Stuby F, Stöckle U (2011) Navigation in surgery of the pelvis and acetabulum: clinical experience, indications and limitations. OP-JOURNAL 27:144–147

Kosmopoulos V, Schizas C (2007) Pedicle screw placement accuracy: a meta-analysis. Spine 32:E111–E120

Lekovic GP, Potts EA, Karahalios DG, Hall G (2007) A comparison of two techniques in image-guided thoracic pedicle screw placement: a retrospective study of 37 patients and 277 pedicle screws. J Neurosurg 7:393–398

Lin YC, Chen CH, Huang HT, Chen JC, Huang PJ, Hung SH, Liu PC, Lee TY, Chen LH, Chang JK (2008) Percutaneous antegrade screwing for anterior column fracture of acetabulum with fluoroscopic-based computerized navigation. Arch Orthop Trauma Surg 128:223–226

Ochs BG, Gonser C, Shiozawa T, Badke A, Weise K, Rolauffs B, Stuby FM (2010) Computer-assisted periacetabular screw placement: Comparison of different fluoroscopy-based navigation procedures with conventional technique. Injury. 41:1297–1305

Rajasekaran S, Vidyadhara S, Shetty AP (2007) Intra-operative Iso-C3D navigation for pedicle screw instrumentation of hangman's fracture: a case report. J Orthop Surg (Hong Kong) 15:73–77

Rammelt S, Gavlik JM, Barthel S, Zwipp H (2002) Value of subtalar arthroscopy in the management of intra-articular calcaneus fractures. Foot Ankle Int 23:706–716

Richter M, Zech S (2011) Navigated retrograde drilling in osteochondrosis dissecans (OCD) of the talus (in German). Oper Orthop Traumatol 23:473–482

Richter M, Geerling J, Zech S, Goesling T, Krettek C (2005) Intraoperative three-dimensional imaging with a motorized mobile C-arm (SIREMOBIL ISO-C-3D) in foot and ankle trauma care: a preliminary report. J Orthop Trauma 19:259–266

Rübberdt A, Feil R, Stengel D, Spranger N, Mutze S, Wich M, Ekkernkamp A (2006) The clinical use of the ISO-C(3D) imaging system in calcaneus fracture surgery. Unfallchirurg 109:112–118

Rübberdt A, Hofbauer VR, Herbort M, Löhrer L, Ochman S, Raschke MJ (2009) 3D navigated osteosynthesis of calcaneal fractures. Open and minimally invasive techniques (in German). Unfallchirurg 112:15–22

Schleicher P, Scholz M, Schnake K et al (2009) Navigation bei thorakolumbalen Wirbelsäulenverletzungen. Trauma Berufskrank 11:100–105

Stöckle U, Schaser K, König B (2007) Image guidance in pelvic and acetabular surgery – expectations, success and limitations. Injury 38:450–462

Tjardes T, Shafizadeh S, Rixen D et al (2010) Image guided spine surgery: state of the art and future directions. Eur Spine J 19:25–45

Watkins 4th RG, Gupta A, Watkins 3rd RG (2010) Cost-effectiveness of image-guided spine surgery. Open Orthop J. 4:228–233

Wendl K, von Recum J, Wentzensen A, Grützner PA (2003) Iso-C (3D-assisted) navigated implantation of pedicle screws in thoracic lumbar vertebrae (in German). Unfallchirurg 106:907–913

Wendl K, Franke J, Grützner PA (2011) Image-guided spine surgery (in German). OP-JOURNAL 27:138-142

Handling Modern Medical Imaging in the High-Tech Operating Theater

Nael Hawi, Musa Citak, Julia Imrecke, Ulrich Lüke, Timo Stübig, Christian Krettek, Tobias Hüfner

The operating room is a central unit in the structure of a hospital. It produces high costs, but in turn generates the highest income. The operating room is a very sensitive and thus stressful working environment and requires staff that is highly qualified. As opposed to aviation, for example, the workflow is more individualized, and especially in trauma surgery it is unpredictable because of emergencies. On top of that, unnecessary stress can be caused by prolonged delays. Arthroscopy and endoscopy have become standard surgical interventions. Thanks to these techniques several other interventions have become more advanced and less invasive. Classically, arthroscopy and endoscopy are used for the bigger joints and for abdominal interventions, for example, cholecystectomy.

19.1 Surgical Set-Up

Since the beginning of the twenty-first century, computer-aided navigation has been used as a standard tool in numerous hospitals (Gebhard et al. 2000; Grutzner et al. 2002; Hofstetter et al. 1999; Nolte et al. 2000). Increased precision has been proved in the field of spinal surgery and during implantation of knee and hip prostheses (Gelalis et al. 2012; Grutzner et al. 2004a, 2004b; Kinzl et al. 2004; Stockl et al. 2004; Kelley et al. 2009). In the field of traumatology, imaging is indispensable. It provides the surgeon with an irreplaceable decision aid. Three-dimensional (3D) C-arm x-ray units have improved imaging quality to such an extent that it almost meets the standard of pre- and postsurgical computer tomography (CT) (Stubig et al. 2009; Geerling et al. 2009; Kendoff et al. 2009; Hüfner et al. 2007; Meier et al. 2005).

However, these technologies are not required for all interventions. The scanning equipment has to be carried in and out of the operating theater, which requires time, occupies space, and promotes wear and tear of the machines. Consequently, the operating theater is a stress-associated environment.

An average operating theater is about 40 m^2 and has a ceiling height of about 3.2 m. Subsequently, the space during complex surgeries is limited. As an example, we present the set-up during spinal endoscopic vertebra replacement:

The patient is positioned in the lateral position. A C-arm x-ray unit and an endoscopy unit are needed with two screens placed opposite each other since the assistant stands facing the surgeon. With the standard devices, two arthroscopy units are needed (◘ Fig. 19.1). At this point, the operating room is filled by up to 60% of its capacity with all the devices and cables needed, which leads to reduced mobility of the C-arm x-ray unit, and potentially unnecessary radiation and frustration can be the result (◘ Fig. 19.1).

Further stress factors have been added in the recent years. The diagnosis-related group (DRG) system that was introduced in 2003 (Hüfner et al. 2007) increased the commercial pressure on hospitals and subsequently on the operating disciplines. It is a fact: In the operating room, money is being earned.

With the introduction of the work-hour regulations for physicians, the pressure continued to increase (Ansorg et al. 2005): The goal is now to perform as many financially lucrative surgeries during a minimum amount of time as possible. This is hard to achieve in maximum-care hospitals.

The total cost for arthroscopy/endoscopy, 3D imaging, and computer-assisted navigation equipment sums up to approximately € 500,000 (in 2012).

On the other hand, the time needed for preparing the devices along with the required maintenance and personnel reduce the time available for performing revenue-generating surgeries (◘ Fig. 19.2).

The introduction of the picture archiving and communication system (PACS) in many medical

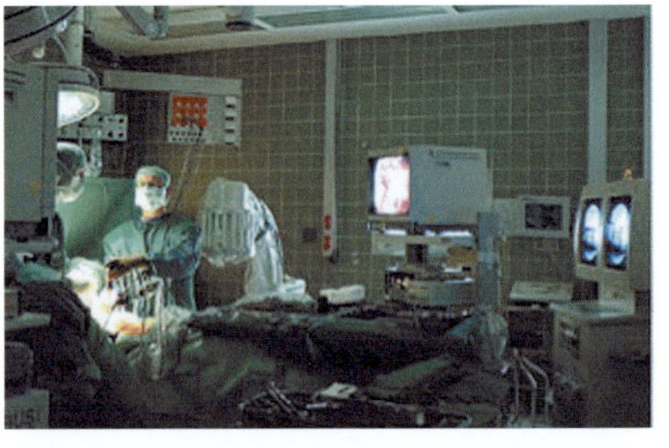

◘ **Fig. 19.1** Endoscopic spinal surgery set-up. Right lateral position. Because of the space taken up by the imaging devices, the operating room is cramped, which could be problematic in emergency situations. (From Hüfner et al. 2012)

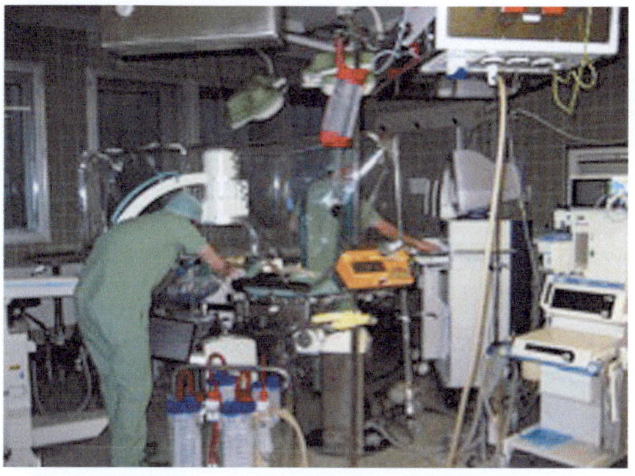

Fig. 19.2 Preparing an operating room for the next surgery. (From Hüfner et al. 2012)

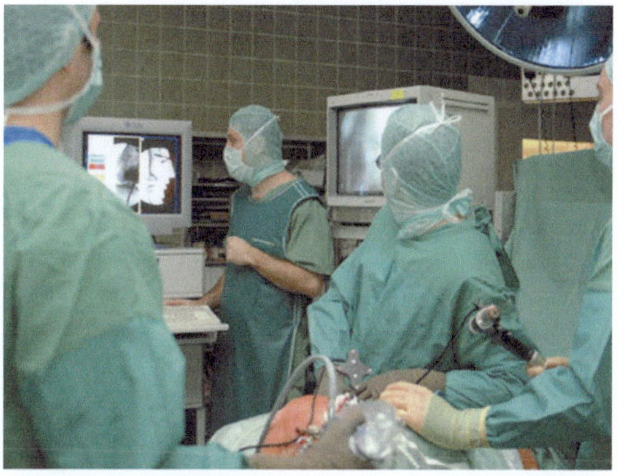

Fig. 19.3 The poor arrangement of the navigation screen leads to the operator's ergonomically unfavorable posture. (From Hüfner et al. 2012)

centers has been valued as an alleviating factor in reducing stress (Frund et al. 2001; Nissen-Meyer et al. 1999; Kondoh et al. 1994; Cannavo 1992). However, this electronic system is developed in cooperation with commercial companies and radiologists and is not usually linked to the surgeon. This means that the images are delivered electronically to the operating room, but not necessarily into the operating field, i.e., close to the operator. Moreover, intraoperatively acquired endoscopic images cannot be easily integrated into the PACS.

Since the early 2000s, many companies have been offering commercial solutions for modern operation room designs depending on the focus of the surgical practice. Endoscopes, intraoperative 3D imaging, navigation, and preoperative imaging and planning are merged into one unit.

The target is to orchestrate the different components in a way that the surgical team is able to review and utilize any needed imaging at any time in an organized and reliable fashion. Hypothetically, this idea of an integrative operating room concept would not only improve ergonomics, but also enable quantification/measurement of time and cost efficiency.

19.2 Methods

In our clinic, we implemented an integrative operating theater concept after extensive analysis (iSuite, Stryker Inc., Duisburg). The core of this system is the endoscopy unit – with a fixed installment and ceiling fixture that is connected to the respective navigation system. To transfer the images, room cameras as well as an in situ camera are part of the system. The server is outside the operating room, and the system and its remote control are operated from the working field of the nursing staff in the operating theater.

The navigation is performed from the operating table itself. The gain of space without the cables is 4 m^2, with cables about 8 m^2, which equals to a gain of about 25%. Because the units are fixed to the ceiling, they can be moved conveniently without needing to rearrange the remaining operating theater furnishings. The operating team can participate in the operation through four freely movable monitors without ergonomic inconveniences (Fig. 19.4).

All units necessary for arthroscopic/endoscopic surgeries are operated via a touchscreen: the high-definition endoscopy camera, the Xenon light source, the water pump, the shaver, and the documentation system (Fig. 19.5).

There are crosslinks to the C-arm and the PACS. Even the preoperative planning can be introduced into the operating room field during the operation utilizing an additional PC station that is also connected to a ceiling monitor.

This operating room system is to be used mainly for arthroscopic and endoscopic procedures. Another focus lies on computer-navigated surgeries, especially on navigated endoscopic knees prosthe-

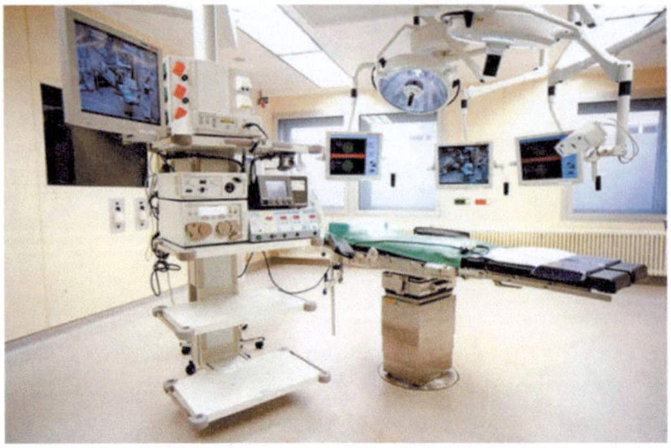

Fig. 19.4 By arranging the units with a ceiling fixation, a cable-free operating room is created allowing for significant space gain. (From Hüfner et al. 2012)

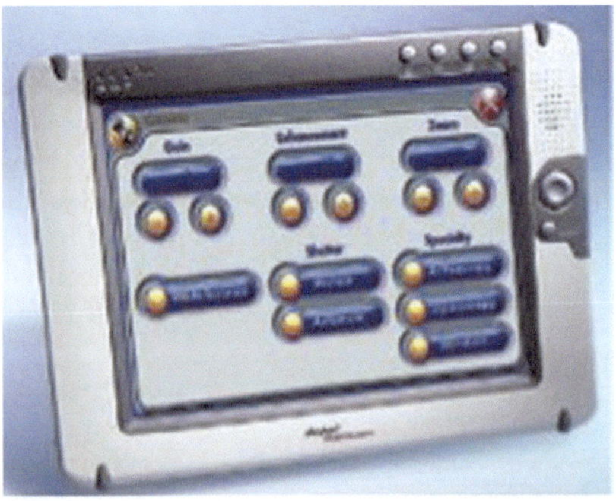

Fig. 19.5 Touch-screen controls are stationed at the non-sterile area to be operated by nursing/assisting staff. (From Hüfner et al. 2012)

ses. In principle, this operating room can also be used for any other surgery that does not specifically require this special equipment.

Potential advantages of this operating room system lie in the improved precision – as a result of the consistent use of the navigation system – the improved ergonomics, and the more efficient workflow. The preparation times are reduced which in turn decreases production costs.

19

19.3 Cost Calculation

The main element when calculating costs is the improved utilization of the core work time during operations by reduction of the warm-up and turn-down times.

The cost of 1 min of operating time is estimated at € 10–30 (Ansorg et al. 2005; Pape et al. 2003). The costs of the previously described operating system were about € 400,000 in 2005 (including remodeling costs), which is around € 50,000/year over 8 years. Assuming costs of € 20 per operation minute, 2,500 operation minutes have to be saved (about 42 h/year). In our own studies, the turnover with a heterogeneous patient population accounts for 30% of the available core work time, which is about 150 min or 2.5 h/day. This turnover time can be estimated at € 10/min, amounting to € 1,500 daily!

19.4 Results

In our own analysis, we were able to perform 112 procedures after installation of the iSuite: 34 knee prostheses, 12 endoscopic spine surgeries, and 66 arthroscopic procedures (28 shoulders, 38 knee reconstructions). We calculated a daily saving of 22–45 min of turnover time, equaling 15–30% of the daily turnover time. Hence, we calculated potential savings of about € 225–450 of the internal costs. This calculation does not yet include the possible additional profit accounted for by the ability of performing more surgeries (made possible by the time savings), and by billing the respective DRG codes.

19.5 Discussion

The proposed operating room system integrates essentially the two elements of trauma/orthopedic surgeries: arthroscopy/endoscopy and computer-aided navigation. An additional essential element, especially in a university hospital setting, is communication via room and in situ cameras and headsets. This also allows for enhanced educational opportunities, since multiple visiting physicians are able to participate interactively with the surgery in an adjacent room. This operating room system enables the live transmission of surgeries and interactive discussions into auditoriums worldwide.

Furthermore, essential time savings can be made by the reduced preparation time and the central documentation system. The improved ergonomics help to maintain an uninterrupted workflow, especially in tertiary centers with high volumes and heterogeneous cases and with highly specialized surgeons/operators.

A commercial operating room concept was evaluated for hard data during a pilot project, paying special attention to time and cost factors. We were able to show that by using this operating theater concept for appropriate surgeries, a daily saving of € 225–450 was achieved.

Further savings were recorded throughout the trial period as follows:

- Persistent usage of the voice operation system, which made waiting for the operating theater assistant unnecessary.
- The sterile calibration of the navigation camera renders the team independent of the presence of the operating theater assistant.
- The C-arm is freely movable thanks to the wireless ceiling installation, which also allows for collision-free movement.

When these factors are included, the estimated time saving is an additional 10–30 min/day, which equals to about € 200–600/day (assuming € 20/min).

The automated imaging transmission through integration of the system with the PACS and Hospital Information System (HIS; *Krankenhaus Informations System*, KIS) makes automated archiving for intraoperative imaging possible. There is no further need to transport data manually or via third-party memory devices, which additionally saves about 15 min/day amounting to € 150 daily.

The time savings hereby add up to 45–90 min daily, equaling about € 575–1,200/day. Hence, profitability is achieved after 42–87 working days/year. This can be exceeded with further efficient usage and higher patient turnover.

This study was a pilot project that was limited by having a study setting. Also, there was no simultaneous control group being evaluated, and ergonomics were not assessed during this pilot phase.

The integrated high-tech operating theater is already in use in many medical centers. The first noncommercial installation was made in 2000 by Regazzoni and Jacob, as an interdisciplinary traumatology and radiology project in Basel (Jacob et al. 2000).

Designing user-friendly technologies is of the essence to increase efficiency and improve ergonomics. The design approach has to be interdisciplinary and has to include all the different disciplines: the surgical department, as well as the anesthesiology, radiology, and nursing staff. The common goal is to optimize the management of resources. This is also necessitated by the budget limitations, and should be part of the early planning stages. Obviously, this is an intricate process and can only be made possible with highly qualified and at the same time motivated staff members.

Since 1994, progress has been achieved in many fields of surgery, for example, the introduction of computer-aided navigation, intraoperative 3D imaging, high-resolution cameras and high-definition screens, along with PACS. For a long time, however, the physical structure of the operating room was incompatible with the installation of these advanced technologies. It is only in the past few years that users and manufacturers of medical equipment have been dedicating time and effort toward the concept of an integrated operating room system.

This is mainly due to the enormous investment that is required to develop a new operating room design, which is only feasible by newly building or completely remodeling an operating room.

The operating room should be designed in an interdisciplinary way to be used by disciplines with requirements for intraoperative imaging. The main surgical disciplines to benefit are:

- Traumatology
- Vascular surgery
- Neurological surgery
- Maxillofacial Surgery
- Ear, nose, and throat surgery

To establish a requirement profile for an interdisciplinary operating room, the different priorities have to be taken into consideration. Because of the magnitude of the investment, the finalization of the concept should be useful and realistic for at least 15 years after completion (Fig. 19.5).

Tab. 19.1 Requirements of different subspecialties for an integrative operating room concept

	Fluoroscopy	Intraoperative 3D C-arm unit	Intraoperative CT	Intraoperative MRI	Ultrasound	Endoscopy/ arthroscopy	Neuromonitoring	Navigation
Traumatology/ orthopedics	++	++	+	–	+	++	–	++
ENT	+	–	+	++	++	++	++	++
Cardiothoracic surgery	+	–	++	+	+	++	++	–
Neurosurgery	++	+	++	++	–	–	++	++

19.6 Commercial Computer-Aided Operating Room Applications

There are multiple approaches by different medical manufacturers that are all following the trend of integrative operating room systems. Many of these manufacturers now offer the integration of multiple products by providing complete application packages that are compatible. Depending on the medical expertise of the manufacturer (endoscopy vs. navigation vs. implants vs. infrastructure vs. video transmission), different solutions are being designed. We list the commercial systems currently available, and the company solution systems are summarized in Tab. 19.1. This listing does not guarantee completeness.

Emphasis on Navigation Brainlab (Heimstetten, Germany). The main focus of BrainSuite lies on navigation, which is shown in its entirety. Additional modular systems include planning and integration of 3D imaging.

Emphasis on Arthroscopy Karl Storz Endoscopes (Tuttlingen, Germany). The operating theater »OR-1« offers, in addition to the arthroscopic instruments, mainly imaging modalities and imaging transmission devices and software. This system also offers the option of integrating a patient tracking system.

Olympus (Hamburg, Germany): EndoALPHA. This manufacturer offers an integrative solution for arthroscopy and video conferences as well as an integrated documentation system.

Richard Wolf (Knittlingen, Germany): CORE. Richard Wolf offers integrated yet modular solutions for endoscopic and arthroscopic surgeries with video transmission.

Smith & Nephew (Marl, Germany): Condor. Smith & Nephew also offer an integrative system for arthroscopies with image processing capabilities.

Emphasis on Modular Infrastructure and Communication Maquet (Rastatt, Germany): AV-Solutions. Besides flexible and modular operating room infrastructures, Maquet offers an audiovisual communication system (AV-Solutions).

S-Cape (Reichenbach, Germany): S-Cape is an integrative solution with a central video processing capability in the operating room. Connection with the KIS/PACS system is also possible for processing and archive imaging.

The magnitude of the investments often lead to difficulties with funding, which becomes critical especially during times of internal service accounting and intragroup cost allocation. The model of Ulm, starting in June 2012, will have to prove that multiple disciplines are able to design and build an operating room system that can be used even for emergencies.

Tab. 19.2 Different solutions to ergonomic and engineering aspects

	Voice control	Touch-panel sterile	Ceiling-bound
Brainlab BrainSuite	–	+	+
Karl Storz OR-1	+	+	+
Maquet AV-Conference	+	+	+
Olympus EndoALPHA	–	+	+
S-Cape Medical Multi-console	–	+	+
Smith & Nephew Condor	+	+	+
Stryker iSuite	+	+	+
Wolf CORE	+	+	+

Tab. 19.3 Connectivity of the different operating room solutions

	Video-conference	Connectivity PACS/KIS	Connectivity of third-party hardware
Brainlab	+	+	+
Karl Storz OR-1	+	+	+
Maquet AV-Conference	+	+	+
Olympus EndoALPHA	+	+	+
S-Cape Medical Multi-console	+	+	+
Smith & Nephew Condor	+			+
Stryker iSuite	+	+	+
Wolf CORE	+	+	+

19.7 Conclusion

There are numerous concepts for the design of operating room focusing on the integration of multiple technology applications (Tab. 19.2, Tab. 19.3). A pilot project was introduced in 2005, which was able to show significant time and cost savings. If an institution is contemplating building such a system, an interdisciplinary use should be considered and implemented in the design process from the very beginning. Even the best technology can only be productive if operated by highly qualified and motivated staff members and by an appropriate management team (Hüfner et al. 2012).

References

Ansorg J, Hassan I, Fendrich V et al (2005) Quality of surgical continuing education in Germany (in German). Dtsch Med Wochenschr 130:508–513

Cannavo M (1992) PACS facts & fallacies. Adm Radiol 11:35–36

Frund R, Techert J, Strotzer M et al (2001) The PACS concept of the University of Regensburg (in German). Rofo 173:362–367

Gebhard F, Kinzl L, Arand M (2000) Limits of CT-based computer navigation in spinal surgery (in German). Unfallchirurg 103:696–701

Geerling J, Kendoff D, Citak M et al (2009) Intraoperative 3D imaging in calcaneal fracture care-clinical implications and decision making. J Trauma 66:768–773

Gelalis ID, Paschos NK, Pakos EEt al (2012) Accuracy of pedicle screw placement: a systematic review of prospective in vivo studies comparing free hand, fluoroscopy guidance and navigation techniques. Eur Spine J 21:247–255

Grutzner PA, Beutler T, Wendl K et al (2002) Computer-assisted screw osteosynthesis of the posterior pelvic ring. Initial experiences with an image reconstruction based optoelectronic navigation system (in German). Unfallchirurg 105:254–260

Grutzner PA, Rose E, Vock B et al (2004a) Intraoperative three-dimensional navigation for pedicle screw placement (in German). Chirurg 75:967–975

Grutzner PA, Zheng G, Langlotz U et al (2004b) C-arm based navigation in total hip arthroplasty-background and clinical experience. Injury 35 [Suppl 1]:A90–95

Hofstetter R, Slomczykowski M, Sati M et al (1999) Fluoroscopy as an imaging means for computer-assisted surgical navigation. Comput Aided Surg 4:65–76

Hüfner T, Citak M, Imrecke J, Krettek C, Stübig T (2012) Handling modern imaging procedures in a high-tech operating room. Unfallchirurg 115:220–225

Hüfner T, Stubig T, Gosling T et al (2007) Cost-benefit analysis of intraoperative 3D imaging (in German). Unfallchirurg 110:14–21

Jacob AL, Regazzoni P, Steinbrich W et al (2000) The multifunctional therapy room of the future: image guidance, interdisciplinarity, integration and impact on patient pathways. Eur Radiol 10:1763–1769

Kelley TC, Swank ML (2009) Role of navigation in total hip arthroplasty. J Bone Joint Surg Am 91 [Suppl 1]:153–158

Kendoff D, Citak M, Gardner MJ et al (2009) Intraoperative 3D imaging: value and consequences in 248 cases. J Trauma 66:232–238

Kinzl L, Gebhard F, Keppler P (2004) Total knee arthroplasty – navigation as the standard (in German). Chirurg 75:976–981

Kondoh H, Ikezoe J, Mori Y et al (1994) PACS in Osaka University Hospital. Comput Methods Programs Biomed 43:57–63

Meier R, Kfuri M Jr, Geerling J et al (2005) Intraoperative three-dimensional imaging with an isocentric mobile C-arm at the wrist (in German). Handchir Mikrochir Plast Chir 37:256–259

Nissen-Meyer S, Reiser M, Adelhard K (1999)PACS. Current status and possible applications (in German). Radiologe 39:255–256

Nolte LP, Slomczykowski MA, Berlemann U et al (2000) A new approach to computer-aided spine surgery: fluoroscopy-based surgical navigation. Eur Spine J 9 [Suppl 1]:S78–88

Pape HC, Grotz M, Schwermann T et al (2003) The development of a model to calculate the cost of care for the severely injured – an initiative of the Trauma Register of the DGU (in German). Unfallchirurg 106:348–357

Stockl B, Nogler M, Rosiek R et al (2004) Navigation improves accuracy of rotational alignment in total knee arthroplasty. Clin Orthop Relat Res 426:180–186

Stubig T, Kendoff D, Citak M et al (2009) Comparative study of different intraoperative 3-D image intensifiers in orthopedic trauma care. J Trauma 66:821–830

Subject Index

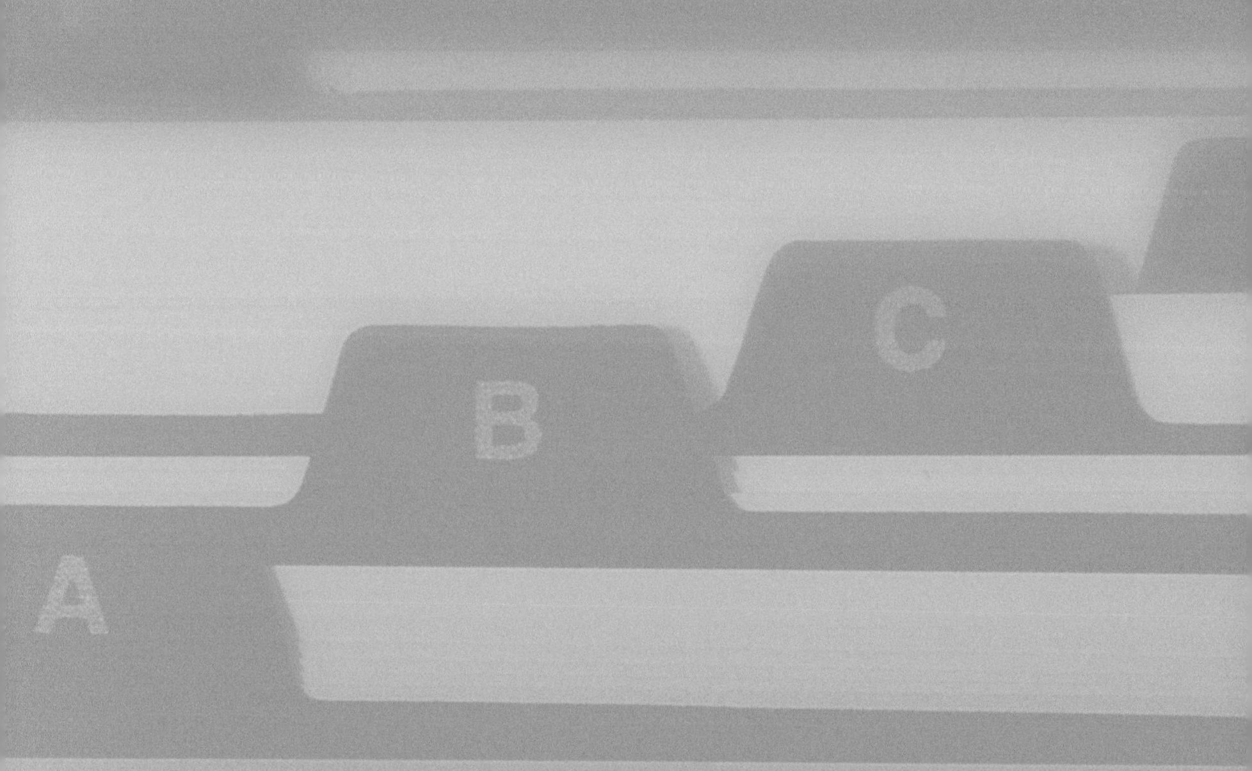

Symbole

A

B

C

D

E

T

U

V

W

Z

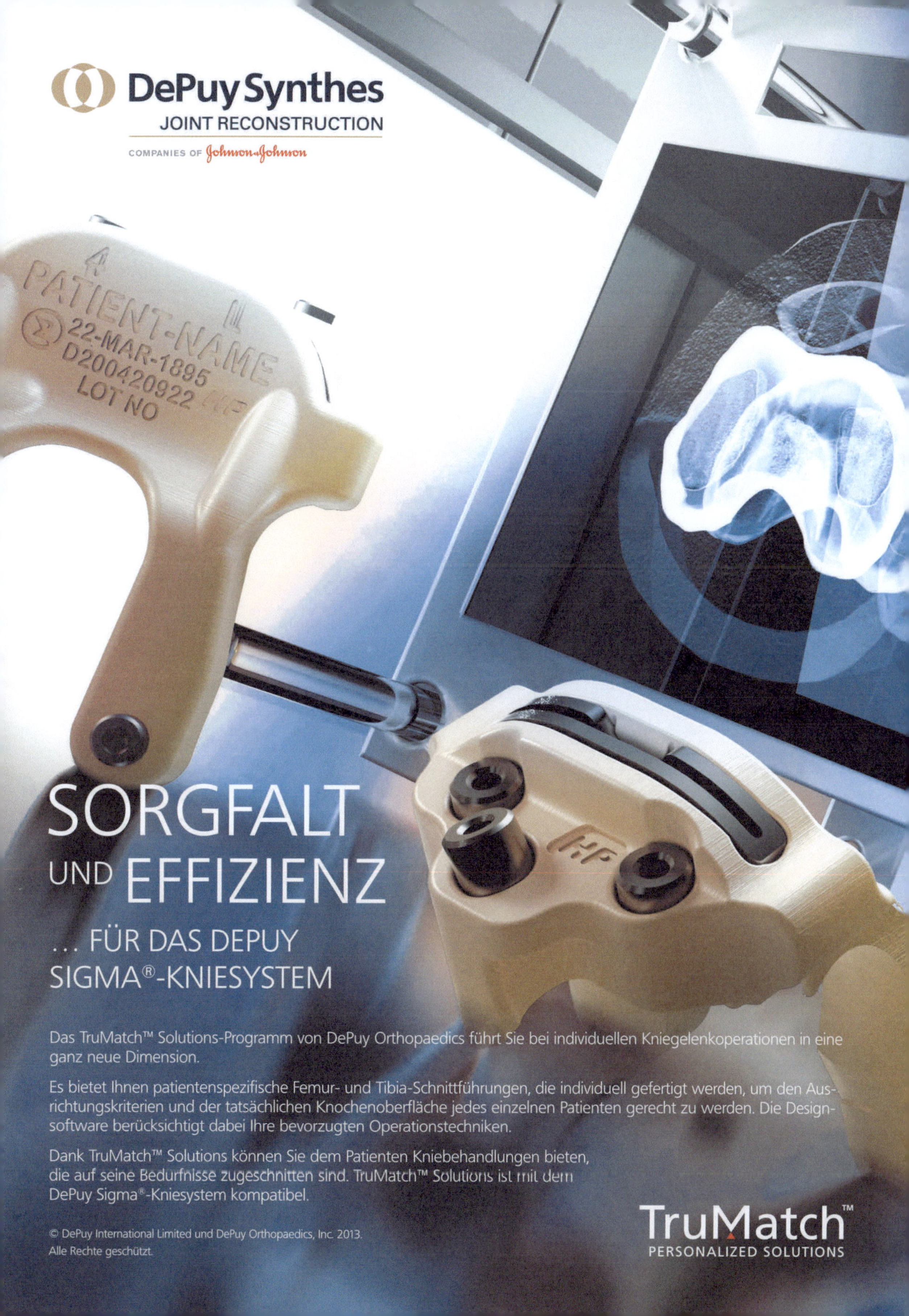
DePuy Synthes
JOINT RECONSTRUCTION
COMPANIES OF Johnson & Johnson
PATIENT-NAME
22-MAR-1895
D200420922
LOT NO
SORGFALT
UND EFFIZIENZ
… FÜR DAS DEPUY
SIGMA®-KNIESYSTEM
Das TruMatch™ Solutions-Programm von DePuy Orthopaedics führt Sie bei individuellen Kniegelenkoperationen in eine ganz neue Dimension.
Es bietet Ihnen patientenspezifische Femur- und Tibia-Schnittführungen, die individuell gefertigt werden, um den Ausrichtungskriterien und der tatsächlichen Knochenoberfläche jedes einzelnen Patienten gerecht zu werden. Die Designsoftware berücksichtigt dabei Ihre bevorzugten Operationstechniken.
Dank TruMatch™ Solutions können Sie dem Patienten Kniebehandlungen bieten, die auf seine Bedürfnisse zugeschnitten sind. TruMatch™ Solutions ist mit dem DePuy Sigma®-Kniesystem kompatibel.
© DePuy International Limited und DePuy Orthopaedics, Inc. 2013.
Alle Rechte geschützt.
TruMatch™
PERSONALIZED SOLUTIONS

MIX
Papier aus verantwortungsvollen Quellen
Paper from responsible sources
FSC® C105338

If you have any concerns about our products,
you can contact us on
ProductSafety@springernature.com

In case Publisher is established outside the EU,
the EU authorized representative is:
Springer Nature Customer Service Center GmbH
Europaplatz 3, 69115 Heidelberg, Germany

Printed by Libri Plureos GmbH
in Hamburg, Germany